The BROKEN BRAIN

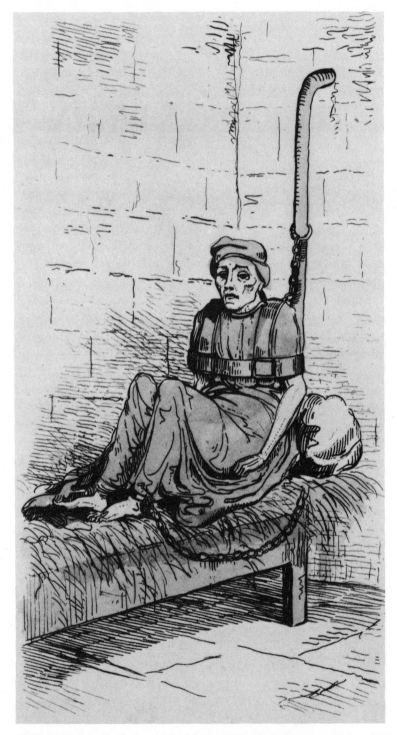

William Norris in chains at Bethlehem Hospital. (Anonymous etching, nineteenth century. *Clements C. Fry Collection. Yale Medical Library*)

The
BROKEN BRAIN

The Biological
Revolution in Psychiatry

by Nancy C. Andreasen, M.D., Ph.D.

1817

HARPER & ROW, PUBLISHERS, New York
Cambridge, Philadelphia, San Francisco,
London, Mexico City, São Paulo, Sydney

In Memoriam:
R.W., S.B., P.P., and E.S.

Grateful acknowledgment is made for permission to reprint:

Figures 11 and 26 from *Principles of Neuroscience,* edited by Eric R. Kandel and James H. Schwartz. Copyright © 1981 by Elsevier Science Publishing Co., Inc. Reprinted by permission of Elsevier Science Publishing Co., Inc. and Eric R. Kandel.

Figure 27 reprinted by permission of the National Library of Medicine.

Excerpt from *The Grapes of Wrath* by John Steinbeck. Copyright 1939, renewed © 1967 by John Steinbeck. Reprinted by permission of Viking Penguin Inc.

Excerpts from *The Poems of Gerard Manley Hopkins,* Fourth Edition, edited by W. H. Gardner and N. H. MacKenzie. 1967: Oxford University Press.

FIRST EDITION

Designed by Ruth Bornschlegel

Library of Congress Cataloging in Publication Data

Andreasen, Nancy C.
   The broken brain.

   Includes index.
   1. Mental illness—Physiological aspects. 2. Neuropsychiatry. I. Title.
RC455.4.B5A53 1984   616.89   83-48782
ISBN 0-06-015281-8

84 85 86 87 88 10 9 8 7 6 5 4 3 2 1

Contents

Acknowledgments

This book tells the story of the relationship between modern brain sciences and psychiatry. That story is moving forward with lightning speed. Even as I was writing in 1983, parts written in 1982 were becoming outdated. I have tried to make the information as current as possible, but the rapid growth of brain science makes that goal impossible to achieve. Our knowledge is simply moving faster than writers and printing presses can present it. Thus this book presents the state of our knowledge more or less as it existed in 1983.

I wish to thank all my patients for the understanding of their illnesses that they have given me over the years, both by sharing their lives with me and by participating in research studies. I wish to thank the many friends and colleagues who assisted in the development of this book by reading parts of the manuscript and offering encouragement, comments, and suggestions. They include Ross Baldessarini, Antonio Damasio, David Dunner, Noble Endicott, I. N. Ferrier, Ralph Giesey, Donald Klein, John Nemiah, Bruce Pfohl, William Preucil, Robert T. Rubin, Edward Sachar, Olivia Stibolt, Mary Ann Volm, Trish Wasek, and George Winokur. My daughter Susan assisted in making the illustrations. The editorial skill of Ted Solotaroff was an invaluable support.

Preface

Although I certainly did not realize it at the time, this book began its gestation along with that of my first child nearly twenty years ago. I was an English professor, a humanist who knew quite a lot about the creative achievements of the human mind but nothing about the human brain and the body from which they derived. The only thing I knew about medicine and doctors was that I wanted to have as little to do with them as possible. However, having the child developing within me, and facing the somewhat frightening prospect of her birth, I found myself becoming curious about how the body works and about how doctors themselves work and think. My life has always been shaped by the Baconian dictum that "knowledge is power." If I knew what was happening and what was going to happen, I would be confident and unafraid.

My doctor was quite sensitive and intelligent, but he did not have time to tell me all that I wanted to know. In retrospect, it is astonishing to me that I was considered an "educated person," and yet I knew absolutely nothing about human biology. The books and pamphlets available to explain the biology of reproduction and the process of delivery tended to be sketchy, and they were also so pompous and paternalistic that I put them down in dismay. I found myself borrowing medical texts from the library of a sympathetic friend who was also a physician. Having some skill in reading other foreign languages, I picked up the medical jargon rather quickly, giving myself a short course in vertebrate embryology, normal physiology, and obstetrics and gynecology. The preparation was not in vain. It turned out that my knowledge helped me through a difficult delivery and permitted me to recognize a potentially fatal postpartum complication that occurred after I was discharged and that required another week in the hospital on IV antibiotics. This experience changed my life. Within the next few months, I decided to become a doctor and a scientist.

I have felt ever since that ordinary readers deserve more-intelligent efforts to translate the world of medicine and science into clear and readable form. Thousands, perhaps millions, of women must have wanted to know the same things that I did. Yet the only choice was between oversimplified and patronizing little pamphlets or the technical and arcane language of medical textbooks. I vowed that eventually

I would try to write something better—the sort of book that I would have liked to read, something that conveyed the truth in both its good and bad aspects and yet avoided confusing and obscurantist jargon.

This book tries to achieve that goal for my own field of specialization, psychiatry. Oddly, although there are thousands of books available about psychology and psychiatry, almost none of them describes this field from the medical perspective. As this book explains, psychiatry is in the process of undergoing a revolutionary change and realigning itself with the mainstream biological traditions of medicine. During the past ten to twenty years, the neurosciences have produced an explosion of knowledge about how the brain works, and this has taught us that many forms of mental illness are due to abnormalities in brain structure or chemistry. Psychiatry is moving from the study of the "troubled mind" to the "broken brain."

Mental illness touches almost all of us in some way. We all have a friend or a child or a parent who has had some type of mental problem. This book was written for the person who wants to know more, who wants the same type of accurate and undiluted information about psychiatry that I was once seeking about obstetrics and gynecology. The need for information is even more imperative in psychiatry. As psychiatry has become more medical and biological, it has become increasingly difficult for ordinary readers (and even for psychiatrists themselves who received their medical training many years ago) to understand. Further, the changes in psychiatry have sweeping social and moral implications. As psychiatry changes to a more biological and medical orientation, attitudes toward mental illness and techniques for treating it will also change.

I began this book with an intent to educate, but while writing it I realized I was also producing a "social manifesto." In addition to making people more educated about psychiatry, I also wanted them to become more enlightened about mental illness. I wanted to teach people to look at the mentally ill as I—or any other reasonably caring psychiatrist—would: as troubled, perplexed human beings who deserve as much sensitivity and love as people who suffer from heart disease, muscular dystrophy, or cancer. As this book explains, the biological revolution in psychiatry has already occurred. It must be followed by a social revolution in the public perception of mental illness.

The BROKEN BRAIN

1

ESCAPING BEDLAM:

Mental Illness in the Past

Now the spirit of the Lord departed from Saul, and an evil spirit from the Lord tormented him. And Saul's servants said to him, "Behold now, an evil spirit from God is tormenting you. Let our Lord now command your servants, who are before you, to seek out a man who is skillful in playing the lyre: and when the evil spirit from God is upon you, he will play it, and you will be well."

—1 SAMUEL 16:14–16

Saul was not the first victim of misunderstanding about the nature of psychiatric illness, nor was he the last. The account of his problems in 1 Samuel is a moving portrayal of a gifted leader who falls prey to depression and despair in an era when such illness was interpreted by sufferer and observer alike as a possession by evil spirits reflecting divine disfavor and when the only treatment available was soothing music.

For centuries people have misunderstood the nature of mental illness. This has led them to react to it with fear, embarrassment, shame, and guilt. They have thought of it as a punishment God gives to sinners, as a spiritual torment due to possession by the devil, or as a moral defect due to weakness of will. In earlier centuries the mentally ill were burned at the stake or pressed to death because they were thought to be possessed. Others were chained in filthy cells for much of their lives, and only a century or two ago people amused themselves by going to observe the inhabitants of Bedlam as if the mentally ill were like animals in a zoo.

The picture on the frontispiece, an anonymous sketch done in 1814, portrays the plight of one such victim. He is an American sailor, William Norris, who was discovered in Bethlehem Asylum (known

1

as "Bedlam") in London by Edward Wakefield, a member of Parliament, in May of 1814. Norris told Wakefield that he was fifty-five years old and that he had been in Bedlam for about fourteen years. He was originally fastened by a single long chain that passed through a hole into the next cell. Because Norris disliked being pulled around by the chain at his keeper's pleasure, he stuffed the chain with straw to keep it from passing through the wall. As a consequence, he was then chained in the manner portrayed on the frontispiece. He had an iron bar around his neck, two iron bars passing over each shoulder, and iron bars holding both arms against his sides. These were connected by a short chain to a pipe on the wall so that he could lie down on his back but could not otherwise move, even to lie on his side. In addition, his leg was also chained to the bed. He had remained chained in this way for more than twelve years.

We wise sophisticates of the 1980s might comfort ourselves with the belief that we live in a more enlightened era. But while it is true that we no longer confine the mentally ill in chains, people who suffer from mental illness are still often the victims of subtler versions of social stigmatization, cruelty, and prejudice. This prejudice grows out of ignorance and misunderstanding about the nature of mental illness. It derives from a failure to realize that mental illness is a physical illness, an illness caused by biological forces and not by moral turpitude.

The following account, based on the case history of an actual patient, shows how a person suffering from mental illness can wear chains just as painful, heavy, and inescapable as those of William Norris. This patient, who died only a few months ago, was killed not by his disease but by the people around him who misunderstood his illness.

> Bill was a curious, witty, sensitive man. He loved Sartre, Sophocles, and Mozart, but was able to defend with equal enthusiasm the virtues of Yeats, Shaw, and Beethoven. By trade he was a pediatrician, and a good one. Mothers recall how he elicited giggles from their children when he could feel popsicles and hamburgers in their stomachs as he was examining them, while children knew intuitively that he was someone whom they could trust with their small bodies and identities. When he died at age forty-five by suicide, many in the community wept at his funeral. No one seemed to understand how it could have happened.

Bill had problems with depression off and on for many years. His first episode occurred when he was twenty, during his junior year at Harvard. He saw a doctor at the student health service and received psychotherapy. It provided very little help, and the depressive symptoms seemed to clear up spontaneously after about six months. He concluded that psychiatry had very little to offer. He continued to feel well for the next four years.

During his senior year in medical school, however, his father died. Bill, who had been very close to his father (also a physician), was plunged into terrible despondency. As a senior medical student, he did not have to attend classes or take examinations, but he did have to work on the hospital wards. He was away for about a month making funeral arrangements, helping his mother, and dealing with his own grief. When he returned to school, he arrived at the wards regularly, but was obviously going about his tasks in a dull, painful manner. One of the residents suggested that he see a psychiatrist. He did, was placed on medication, and improved slowly. Nevertheless, because of the mixture of grief and depression, he had a rather protracted period of despondency that lasted about four months. As a consequence, the Promotions Committee of the medical school decided that he should not be permitted to graduate. Because of his problem with mental illness, they indicated to him that he would be required to remain in school for another year, essentially repeating his senior year. If he were symptom-free during this time period, they would then permit him to graduate. He did so, quietly holding his feelings of humiliation and despair within himself. Doctors, he had been told, have a great responsibility for the lives of other people. The medical school could not permit him to graduate unless it was sure he would be able to uphold this responsibility.

Because his graduation was held back, he had some difficulty in becoming accepted into an internship and residency, in spite of the fact that he graduated from Harvard magna cum laude and earned many honors during medical school. Hospitals were reluctant to accept doctors who might have a problem with mental illness. Nevertheless, he eventually obtained an internship and residency at a good university hospital in the Midwest. During this time, he married a woman whom he had known since his undergraduate years at Harvard with whom he shared many interests. After completing his residency, he went into private practice, and she obtained a job as a school music teacher. Two daughters were born to them during the next several years. During this time, Bill experienced another episode of depression, which was again treated with medication and cleared up within a month. Because he had already been sensitized to the risks of being stereotyped as mentally ill, he chose to see a psychiatrist in a neighboring community fifty miles away. He felt tempted to prescribe medication for himself, since this would prevent anyone from knowing about his problem, but he knew it was ethically wrong, as well as unwise.

Things remained relatively tranquil until Bill was thirty-five. One day at breakfast he noticed that his wife's skin had a rather sallow color. She had also been complaining of excessive tiredness. Within the next several days her skin turned saffron. She was hospitalized, evaluated, and found to have inoperable cancer of the liver. During the next year Bill watched her decline and die. Their children were two and four at the time. As he watched her die, he struggled with grief, anger, frustration, and fear. He was soon going to lose someone whom he loved, the perfect person with whom to share his life. He wondered if he would be able to cope without her, managing a home, children, and his practice. He began to feel a return of the old feelings of despair and despondency, but he fought them off, knowing that he had to be as strong as possible in order to help her and the two girls. Two months before her death, he had several outbursts of uncontrollable weeping while at work. He felt this was unacceptable, saw his doctor in the neighboring community, and was hospitalized in a psychiatric facility for one month. His wife, battling with her own feelings of loss and despair, could not quite forgive him for deserting her when she needed him during the final months of her life. Some people in the community had trouble understanding why he could not maintain better control of himself. They thought him weak and lacking in self-discipline.

After the funeral, Bill threw himself into his practice. He found a dependable older woman to care for his children, and life seemed reasonably comfortable, although a bit lonely. About a year after Mary's death, Bill began to date. He sensed instinctively that he was not suited for a bachelor's existence, even with a good person available to help with the two girls. He missed discussing the day's events over dinner and making plans for the future with another person who seemed to care. He eventually married a nurse, ten years younger than he, who had been divorced once before. Unlike Mary, she was unintellectual, lighthearted, and fun-loving. Bill thought she would provide a healthy balance to his own somewhat graver approach to life, and it seemed good that she was distinctly different from Mary.

During the first year or two after their marriage, all went well. Joann seemed to enjoy the two girls almost as if she were their mother. Bill tried to share her interest in sports events and barhopping, even though he might have preferred to read a book, listen to classical music, or watch a vintage movie on TV. Shortly after Joann turned thirty, however, she expressed some discomfort with the relationship. She said that she felt confined by monogamy and wanted to try having an open marriage. Bill did not like the idea, but eventually acquiesced. They agreed that Joann could go out wherever she pleased three nights a week with no questions asked, and that he would be free to go out the other three nights, while they would spend Sunday evenings together. Bill made one desultory attempt to have an affair, and thereafter spent his three evenings quietly at home. He began to feel steadily more enraged, however, when he watched Joann leave at 7:00 and return home at 1:00 or 2:00 A.M. He again began to develop symptoms of depression and sought treatment for them. After talking the situation over with his psychiatrist, he decided to tell Joann that they must return to a monogamous relationship. After thinking the proposal over for about a month, Joann decided instead that she wanted a divorce. Marriage, she said, just wasn't fun anymore. She was getting older and felt her youth might be slipping away from her. She did not want to have her thirties spoiled by lack of freedom and the responsibilities of a husband and two daughters.

So, for the second time, Bill found that he had lost a wife. It was the third time he had lost a loved one. Making matters worse, Joann continued to live in the same community, and he could not avoid running into her with her various boyfriends from time to time. One night he saw her at a local restaurant, felt the mixture of love and hatred with which he had been struggling ever since she left him, and went home to console himself by having several drinks. Bill typically did not imbibe more than an occasional beer on weekends, and so four ounces of scotch quickly disinhibited him. He got back in his car, drove past her apartment, and stopped outside. He went up to the door, began knocking on it, and asked to talk with her. She opened the door slightly but refused to let him in, finally slamming the door in his face. He concluded she must be inside with a boyfriend and was overwhelmed with rage. He started pounding on the door. Joann called the police. Bill found himself arrested for public intoxication and saw his name in headlines in the local newspaper. He was mortified.

During the six months since Joann had left him, he had been

having symptoms of depression and seeing his doctor for them. He had felt so bad that he had had to miss several days of work, but he tried very hard to cope. After his arrest and its bad publicity, he went to pieces. Other physicians in the community knew that he had been having problems, but no one made any attempt to offer help or sympathy. Some thought he simply needed to be tougher, while others thought he was behaving irresponsibly. Having put most of his energy into his work and his family, Bill had few close friends. The two or three whom he did have held back from approaching him because of uncertainty or embarrassment. After about a week of feeling so bad that he was unable to go into the office, Bill decided he must reenter the hospital. Bill's depressive symptoms did not improve after three weeks on medication, and so he was treated with electroconvulsive therapy (ECT). This helped a great deal, and Bill was able to leave the hospital after a total of six weeks, planning to return to work in another week or two.

When he returned home, however, he learned that the state medical examiners had decided to temporarily suspend his license because of his recent psychiatric hospitalization. Bill went to the state capitol to appeal his case and was upheld. Again, however, the story was picked up in the newspapers, and Bill saw his name in headlines and even heard himself discussed on TV. His children, now of school age, began to ask their father what he had done wrong. Naturally, he found this difficult to explain.

Two weeks after his medical license was reinstated, he took his life unexpectedly. He had just seen his doctor the previous week and although he expressed anger and frustration about the bad publicity he had received, overall he indicated that he was feeling back to his usual self and was looking forward to returning to work. Although still confronted with many problems, such as the responsibility of being a single parent for two young children and community disapproval of his recent divorce (Bill was too much of a gentleman to tell the real story), he was confident that he would be able to cope.

Bill left no suicide note, so one can only speculate on what precisely had happened. A reasonable guess is that he felt terribly lonely and isolated, rejected by friends and community, and tormented by gnawings of failure and inadequacy. His profession had told him directly that signs of weakness could not be tolerated and that mental illness is a sign of weakness He must have thought that he was becoming depressed again and that he might require rehospitalization. If that were to happen, this time his license might really be revoked. Then he would have lost his career as well, not to mention any means of supporting his children. If he were to die, they would at least have his life insurance, which was substantial. He did not dare to discuss his suicidal thoughts with his doctor, who would have insisted he return to the hospital.

If Bill had not had to feel guilty about his episodes of mental illness or to worry about the professional and social consequences of seeking treatment, he would almost certainly still be alive. He was as encaged by his illness as William Norris was by his iron bars and chains. What is worse, Bill's illness—depression—almost always responds well to treatment. Bill had always recovered relatively quickly in the past, and undoubtedly he would have again if society had not suggested that he would be penalized for admitting that he was ill and seeking treatment again.

If Bill had needed chemotherapy for cancer, he would have been surrounded by compassionate friends and colleagues. If he had needed hospitalization for coronary bypass surgery, his room would have been full of flowers. Because he had mental illness, people pulled away, avoided him, or even disdained him. The flowers that should have been sent to his hospital room were sent to his funeral instead. Had he received some genuine support from even four or five of the thousand people who appeared there, he probably would have felt enough hope and attachment to push through the spot of darkness and isolation in which he found himself and reach the light beyond.

People can ill afford to pull away from mental illness or remain ignorant about it, for it affects the life of nearly everyone. It is perhaps the commonest type of illness occurring in our society. It is estimated that half the patients who see family practitioners are suffering from some type of psychiatric problem. Nearly everyone knows a person who has suffered from serious mental illness requiring hospitalization or treatment. Many people have seen what a serious mental illness can do to upset family relationships. Many have seen promising young people become devastated for the remainder of their lives after an illness such as schizophrenia strikes them in their early teens or twenties. Many, in fact, have experienced mental illness in their own families, and have hungered for more precise information about how it was caused, how it can best be treated, whether it is curable, and whether it is hereditary. Many have experienced mild suggestions of mental illness in themselves, moments of hopelessness or depression that seem overwhelming but lift spontaneously. They look at the victims of more prolonged and serious illnesses and see a fine line between their own experiences and serious mental illness, wondering if someday they too might break down completely.

The extent to which mental illness affects the lives of nearly everyone leads to ambivalent feelings. On the one hand, people are genuinely curious to learn more and to understand. On the other hand, they are frightened and embarrassed, and the fear and embarrassment lead them to ignore, to deny, and even to dislike anything pertaining to psychiatry. For many people, "You need to see a shrink" is still the ultimate insult.

Hostile and critical attitudes toward the mentally ill can change only through increased understanding and knowledge. The change will be speeded up further if people have an opportunity to learn about the transformations that have been occurring in psychiatry during the past ten to twenty years. Psychiatry, like the prodigal son, has returned home to its place as a specialty within the field of medicine. It has become increasingly scientific and biological in its orientation. Psychiatry now recognizes that the serious mental illnesses are *diseases* in the same sense that cancer or high blood pressure are diseases. Mental illnesses are diseases that affect the brain, which is an organ of the body just as the heart or stomach is. People who suffer from mental illness suffer from a *sick or broken brain,* not from weak will, laziness, bad character, or bad upbringing.

The recognition that mental illnesses are diseases affecting the brain is the basis of the biological revolution in psychiatry. This teaching has already done a great deal to diminish the fear, shame, and guilt attached to mental illness. As the public grows to understand its implications better, we should enter a new era of genuine enlightenment concerning the nature of mental illness. Its victims and their friends and relatives will understand its nature and causes and be able to discuss them without shame and embarrassment.

This book was written because of a belief that people would like to have accurate information about the nature of mental illness; and that if they had accurate information, they could relate to the mentally ill with greater compassion, understanding, and patience. It is filled with facts about the dramatic changes that have been occurring in psychiatry and the related neurosciences during the past ten to twenty years. It begins by describing the historical factors in America that delayed widespread acceptance of psychiatry as a branch of medicine specializing in diseases of the brain. The biological approach to psychiatry, which began in Europe, has been very late in arriving in this country. Later chapters explain how the biological revolution will affect the way we think about mental illness, the search for its causes, and the treatment that patients receive.

Although the improved understanding of mental illness cannot help Bill, it will do much to help others.

2

THE "BIOLOGICAL REVOLUTION" IN PSYCHIATRY:

How Did It Begin?

Every fool reads what his teachers tell him, and calls his credulity science or morality as confidently as his father called it divine revelation.

—GEORGE BERNARD SHAW,
The Revolutionist's Handbook,
Man and Superman

The stereotypes of the psychiatrist are multiple. One is of a bearded man who smokes a pipe, listens carefully and nods knowingly, and occasionally makes an insightful or perceptive comment. He conveys the impression that he is omniscient and can read your mind. His office contains a couch, and the patient may lie down and talk about his early childhood. Eventually the patient may be helped by this cathartic process. But it is very expensive and seems to take a very long time.

An alternate stereotype is that the psychiatrist is a little crazy himself. This one complements his beard with longer hair, dresses somewhat unconventionally, and seems interested in expressing his own individuality. He is interested in helping people to expand their minds and to achieve self-realization and self-actualization. He too uses the techniques of psychotherapy as his principal tools, and may also emphasize various forms of group therapy. One would worry a bit before taking one's son, daughter, husband, or wife to this therapist, but he may be helpful to swinging singles.

A third stereotype is of the psychiatrist as punitive and coercive. He is a person who may lock you up in a cuckoo's nest if you tell him too much, or even if you don't. This psychiatrist dispenses both psychotherapy and physical treatments. The physical treatments are perceived as violent and destructive rather than helpful—shock therapies, lobotomy, and mind-numbing drugs.

Like most stereotypes, these are of course oversimplifications: Most psychiatrists are ordinary people, preoccupied during their off-hours with weeds, diets, and the problems of rearing and educating their children. But these stereotypes point to a common, important, and *outdated* misconception about the nature and role of psychiatry. Most people perceive the psychiatrist as a person who principally dispenses psychotherapy. Drug therapies are used occasionally, but only for the really sick and dangerous. One might be willing to go to a psychiatrist to talk and listen, but if he pulls out a prescription pad, something must be awfully wrong.

These particular stereotypes of psychiatry are to some extent peculiarly American. They derive from the fact that Freudian psychodynamic theories became widely accepted in our country during the early twentieth century as they did in no other. To most Americans the word *psychiatry* is nearly synonymous with *psychoanalysis.* Many Americans are even confused about whether psychiatrists are actually medical doctors. In fact, psychoanalysis is one perspective within the general field of psychiatry. Throughout most of the rest of the world, it occupies a relatively minor position and is used primarily to treat people who are mildly ill, particularly those who are among the economic and social elite. In Europe and the developing nations, psychiatry is predominantly biological and medical. The origins of psychiatry, as well as its sister discipline, neurology, are clearly biological.

Vienna and Boston: Around 1910

In 1910 Sigmund Freud made a visit to the New World. For him it was a great personal triumph after many years of frustration. On this visit he delivered a series of lectures on psychoanalysis to an audience of physicians and psychologists from the Boston area at Clark University in Worcester, Massachusetts. The response was intoxicating for lecturer and audience alike. When Freud had introduced his ideas to conservative Viennese medical societies, he was greeted with skepticism and doubt. In fact, he was sometimes the victim of mockery and even hatred. But while Europeans had their reservations, Freudian psychoanalysis enchanted Americans. Freudian theories were original, creative, interesting, insightful, logical, and liberating. Americans have always loved new ideas and new technologies. Freud offered them a new theory of the mind and a new technology for unlocking its secrets.

The revolution that began in Boston in 1910 slowly spread across the country. In New York, Chicago, San Francisco, and every other major and minor city, major and minor psychoanalytic institutes or training centers were created. By the 1940s, psychoanalysis dominated American thinking in psychiatry. Psychoanalytic psychotherapy for a time became nearly synonymous with the treatment of mental and emotional problems.

Freud, of course, was pleased to see his ideas so widely accepted. But he would probably be a bit puzzled and chagrined by the reverent dogmatism that his theories have sometimes achieved during recent years, particularly in America. For Freud began his work hoping to understand and to map the brain rather than the mind. His early training was as a researcher in the brain sciences, or what in more recent years has been called "neuroscience." He was a gifted student of the leading brain researchers and neurologists of his time, men such as Brücke, Meynert, and Charcot. When he was a medical student and resident physician, the neurosciences were filled with an air of excitement much as they are today. The great neurologists Broca and Wernicke had proved that the brain contained specific areas that controlled different functions, such as the ability to speak, and that damage to different tiny areas within a larger specific area could cause different kinds of damaged language functions. Injuries that occurred in the front (in "Broca's area") left a person nearly mute, but able to understand everything that was said to him, while injuries that were further back (in "Wernicke's area") left the person speaking fluent nonsense and unable to understand the speech of others. Golgi was developing new staining techniques so that brain cells could be seen more clearly under the microscope; fiber tracts connecting different parts of the brain were being traced; and the effects of electrical stimulation of the brain were being studied.

Freud wanted desperately to share in this exciting research, and to obtain a university position that would permit him to explore the brain sciences. He was prevented by anti-Semitism and lack of independent means. His Jewishness made an academic appointment unlikely, and his need to earn a living and to support a family drove him into private practice. One of his earliest published works, however, was a treatise on aphasia (loss of the ability to communicate in words), placing him squarely in the tradition of the brain research of his era. (Ironically, this book is not included in the twenty-four-volume set of Freud's *Complete Psychological Works.*)

Once in private practice, with the technology of university laboratories closed to him, Freud applied his curiosity about the workings of the human brain to understanding the maladies that his patients experienced. Because of his prior training in neuroscience, his medical practice included many patients with neurological complaints. They were often wealthy Viennese ladies seeking help for peculiar paralyses and pains. Freud soon realized that most of these complaints had no organic basis, but were instead due to neuroses. No obvious treatments were available, because no obvious cause could be found.

Like any good doctor seeking to help his patients, Freud experimented with a variety of approaches. One of these, hypnosis, enjoyed some popularity at the time. Freud had learned this technique from two skilled French physicians, Liébault and Bernheim. He also experimented with another technique, having the patient talk at random about early experiences (or "chimney sweeping"), a technique that had been developed by one of his friends, Josef Breuer, who had used it to treat several patients seen in his medical practice. They discovered that it seemed to help, and they reported the result to their colleagues. To many, Freud and Breuer appeared to be on the lunatic fringe. Breuer soon gave up the technique, but Freud persisted, and in so doing discovered many interesting patterns of human thinking and behavior—the meanings hidden in the unconscious life of dreams, the sexual attraction that young children feel toward parents of the opposite sex, the jealousy they feel toward parents of the same sex, the traumatic effects that early life events may have. He found that fantasies reflect unfulfilled wishes, and that making the unconscious conscious may help people change pathological behavior. Through these discoveries the new science of psychoanalysis was born. As we have seen, its widest acceptance was in the United States.

Munich: 1903–26

Meanwhile, in Europe the neuroscientists, neurologists, and psychiatrists continued their work. Simultaneously with Freud's development of psychoanalytic theories concerning the functions of the mind, the scientists within the university laboratories from which Freud had been excluded continued to describe and map the structure of the brain. Clinicians working with seriously ill patients began to develop improved definitions of their illnesses and even to discover their causes. Perhaps the greatest rival to Sigmund Freud was a man whose name few Americans would even recognize: Emil Kraepelin. While Freud was creating the psychoanalytic movement, Kraepelin was laying the foundations for another development, the modern biological revolution in psychiatry.

Emil Kraepelin was a professor at several different medical schools in Germany and culminated his career by becoming head of the Department of Psychiatry in Munich. When Kraepelin began his work in the late nineteenth century, the exciting descriptions of Wernicke and Broca concerning the localization of brain functions and the classification of language disorders had just been completed. Psychiatry, a sister discipline to neurology (and often not even distinguished from it), seemed capable of similar discoveries.

In Munich, Kraepelin assembled some of the best minds available to do research in neuroscience. As in the case of Kraepelin, most of their names are unfamiliar to people not trained in medicine. Even within medicine, at least in America, the members of Kraepelin's Department of Psychiatry are thought of as neurologists rather than as psychiatrists because of their interest in brain structure and function. Alzheimer, for example, devoted his career to studying illnesses leading to dementia, and eventually identified "Alzheimer's disease," perhaps the most common form of senility. It is characterized and defined by specific kinds of changes in brain cells that Alzheimer identified under the microscope.

The discoveries of clinicians like Alzheimer were facilitated by the work of more basic researchers in the department, men like Nissl and Brodmann. Nissl is famous for developing a staining technique that permits brain cells to be seen more clearly under the microscope. Brodmann is famous for using Nissl's method of staining to show that different parts of the brain are highly specialized and contain different kinds of nerve cells, paving the way for more recent discoveries that different parts of the brain contain different abilities.

For most of the world, Kraepelin's department in Munich represented mainstream psychiatry. The work of Freud was either a minor tributary or a diversion into a quiet and somewhat restricted estuary.

Kraepelin's own contribution to psychiatry was to describe and identify different specific types of major psychiatric illnesses. At the time he began his work, confusion prevailed. If one were to walk into a psychiatric ward in the nineteenth century, one would find it filled with very sick patients being treated by doctors equally perplexed about the nature of their diagnoses, the causes and likely outcomes of their illnesses, and the best possible treatments. A patient who wandered around excitedly mumbling to himself might be called a case of "delirious mania," but no one knew precisely what that meant. Another, who spoke constantly of the fact that he was Napoleon, escaped from Elba and living in Paris, might be called a case of "dementia paranoides," but again, no one knew clearly what that meant. Descriptive names were applied, but they were not very helpful to clinicians. As long as no one knew which patients had similar disorders and which disorders had a similar outcome, it was impossible to make any useful predictions about the future.

In medicine, the primary purpose of defining and diagnosing specific illnesses in particular patients is to be able to make useful predictions. Ideally, when a doctor makes a diagnosis, he is also making a series of statements about the future: that the patient with that diagnosis will eventually recover fully rather than deteriorate and die; that the patient will respond to a particular type of medication; that the patient's children will have a 50-percent chance of developing the illness as well; or that others around the patient may "catch" the disease.

When Kraepelin began his work, no one even knew what the diseases were that psychiatrists were treating. Kraepelin laid the foundations of modern biological psychiatry by identifying some of these specific diseases. His approach was that of the good empirical scientist: He observed patients carefully, studied their symptoms, described these symptoms in detail, and followed his patients over the course of several years. When he did this, he made an amazing discovery, a discovery whose simplicity characterizes much of great science: Some patients who had a specific set of symptoms recovered spontaneously with minimal treatment, while other patients rarely recovered, usually deteriorated, and required lifetime institutionalization. He further discovered that the patients who recovered tended to have symptoms of either euphoria and increased energy or depression and decreased energy. He placed these patients together in a single group because they had a similar outcome in spite of their diverse symptoms, and he called their illness *manic-depressive insanity.* The second group of patients that he identified were people who became ill at a relatively young age, suffered from many different kinds of symptoms (delusions, hallucinations, excitement, confusion, depression, elation), and tended to deteriorate slowly and inexorably over the course of time so that they became completely incapacitated. He named their illness *dementia praecox*—*dementia* referring to the characteristic deterioration, and *praecox* to the early age of onset. (A few years later, a Swiss psychiatrist, Eugen Bleuler, renamed the illness *schizophrenia.*)

Kraepelin's recognition of these two illnesses within the confusing array of patients living in the nineteenth- and early twentieth-century psychiatric hospitals laid the foundations of modern psychiatry. He described these illnesses, as well as a number of others that he also defined, in a series of textbooks that he wrote and rewrote between 1883 and 1926. In these texts he provided careful descriptions of symptoms, clear case histories, and a thoughtful discussion of possible causes of major mental illnesses. In every country except the United States, Kraepelin, not Freud, is regarded as the founding father of modern psychiatry.

Kraepelin did not attempt to map the topography of the mind, as Freud did. He was not interested in mild illnesses such as the neuroses, as Freud was. He was not preoccupied with helping the essentially healthy become happier and freer, as were many of Freud's disciples. He saw himself as a professor of medicine who specialized in major mental disorders. From this perspective, he viewed these disorders as illnesses that were probably caused by some as yet unrecognized physical factors, such as infection or degenerative brain diseases. Most of the discoveries of modern psychiatry represent a series of footnotes to and amplifications of Kraepelin's textbooks.

Baltimore: 1913

In America, however, Freudian psychoanalysis prevailed over Kraepelinian biological psychiatry. Further, another tradition, particularly American, was soon added: the behavioral approach. Behaviorism has its intellectual roots in British empiricism. Its scientific roots perhaps began with the Russian Pavlovian school's physiological research on various reflexes. But it also began early in the United States and contributed a special set of attitudes and ideas to American psychiatry that tended to further impede the acceptance of Kraepelinian biological psychiatry.

Behaviorism was founded in America by John B. Watson not long after Freud visited this country to give his series of lectures at Clark University. Watson's famous paper, *Psychology as the Behaviorist Views It,* was published in 1913. His most influential followers have been Clark Hull and B. F. Skinner. Like Freud and Kraepelin, these behaviorists had a vastly ambitious goal. While Freud hoped to map the functions of the mind, and Kraepelin the abnormalities of the brain, Watson, Hull, and Skinner hoped to map the general laws governing human behavior.

The behaviorists began their work because of frustration with the imprecision and ambiguity that characterized thinking about the human mind and the way people behave. They quickly took a firm antithetical stance toward most of Freud's methods and teachings. While Freud and his followers worked by listening to their patients describe past experiences and feelings, the behaviorists argued against the value of introspection and the validity of subjective experiences. They believed that the proper way to study how human beings think and feel is through studying what they *do.* Behavior, not ideas or emotions, is the proper province of psychology.

The difference between the psychoanalytic approach of Freud and the behavioral approach of Watson is vividly illustrated in two famous case histories, the case of "Little Hans" and the case of "Little Albert." Little Hans was a five-year-old boy whose father consulted Dr. Freud for treatment of the child's irrational fear that he would be bitten by a horse. Hans's first symptom was an attack of severe anxiety while out on the street. Later he expressed a more specific phobia, a fear of horses. Little Hans's parents were determined from the beginning that he not be laughed at or bullied because of this phobia, and they went to Dr. Freud in order to relieve his symptoms through psychoanalysis.

The analysis was carried out indirectly with considerable assistance from Little Hans's father. The major goal was to release the repressed wishes and conflicts that were causing the phobia. As it turned out, Little Hans was suffering from a variety of repressed fears, sexual drives, and aggressive instincts. He was fearful of castration; jealous of his baby sister, who was born when he was three and a half; and, above all, felt threatened by his omnipotent and powerful father. Because all these feelings were unacceptable to his consciousness, he repressed them, but they later came out expressed as an irrational fear of being bitten by a horse. In this instance, the boy's fear and anxiety concerning his father were displaced onto a horse. The process of analysis involved having Freud and Hans's father help the boy understand the displaced fear and release it through playful behavior, such as biting his father when they were roughhousing.

The case of "Little Hans" was published in 1909. Depending on one's point of view, it is either an intellectual *tour de force,* full of well-written and insightful observations about infantile sexuality and child rearing, or it is an example of how fanciful a scientist can become when he indulges in theoretical speculation on the basis of very little evidence.

John B. Watson held the latter point of view. The case of "Little Albert" was described by Watson and Rayner in 1920. This case report was intended to represent the antithesis of the Freudian psychodynamic approach. Little Albert did not seek the treatment of an eminent doctor for an inexplicable and crippling fear; rather, he was a small boy who was taught to fear by a group of experimental psychologists working in a research laboratory and trying to map the laws governing human behavior.

Watson and Rayner were interested in the effects of conditioning, particularly in how the reaction to one stimulus can generalize to other stimuli. Little Albert began with an innate fear of loud noises. In the laboratory of Watson and Rayner, he displayed fear when a noise was made behind him by striking an iron bar. Watson and Rayner then made the identical noise just as the boy reached out to touch a rat, which he had previously found amusing and interesting. His original fear of loud noises was soon transferred to the rat because the two stimuli were now related to one another. Eventually, through the process of stimulus generalization, he also became afraid of other furry objects. Thus, like little Hans, little Albert now had an animal phobia. This phobia, however, was not caused by repressed unconscious fears and desires, but rather by behavioral conditioning. He had a natural fear of loud noises. He was then taught to fear rats as well when the two stimuli of loud noises and rats were paired. From the point of view of Watson and Rayner, this is the way such phobias typically develop. They are best treated, not through recovery of unconscious material, but rather through deconditioning.

Because it is both easier and more humane to experiment with animals, much of the research of the behaviorists has begun with animal models. The "Skinner Box," in which rats are observed responding to a variety of stimuli and situations, has become a symbol of behavioral research, just as the human patient free-associating on the couch has become a symbol of psychodynamic research. Traditional behavioral research emphasizes objective observation with careful control of the experimental situation.

Opponents objected that this type of research was arid and superficial, neither interesting nor generalizable to the complex conditions of human interactions. Psychiatrists, who were becoming principally psychoanalytically oriented, rarely bothered to pay close attention to behavioral theories and research; when they did, they frequently objected that the work of the behaviorists was of little help in understanding abnormal behavior and that its "black box" approach was mechanistic, oversimplified, and even inhumane. But the defenders of behaviorism continued to insist on the value of their approach. Its building blocks were simple, elegant experiments. Any of these alone might seem superficial or of little value in understanding the complexities of human behavior, but taken together, a large enough series of these experiments might be used to explain all aspects of human behavior. Because these experiments were objective and precise, because they were based on careful scientific design, and because they drew on a large sampling of behavior rather than single case studies, they would ultimately build an imposing scientific edifice that would stand the test of time.

Freud, Kraepelin, and Watson are the prototypes for three quite different points of view concerning the understanding and treatment of mental illness. Historically, the psychodynamic and behavioral points of view have dominated American thinking, while European thinking has been influenced by all but has been predominantly biological or Kraepelinian. However, in America in the 1980s, the balance between these points of view has begun to shift. The emphasis is swinging, and swinging quite strongly, toward a biological model.

3

COMPETING MODELS OF MENTAL ILLNESS:

Psychodynamic, Behavioral, and Biological

The Brain, within its Groove
Runs evenly and true—
But let a splinter swerve—
'Twere easier for You—

To put a Current back
When Floods have slipped the Hills—
And scooped a Turnpike for Themselves—
And trodden out the Mills—

—EMILY DICKINSON, *No. 556*

Freud, Kraepelin, and Watson represent three competing models of how mental illnesses are caused, how they should be defined and studied, and how they should be treated. These are the psychodynamic (or psychoanalytic) model, the biological (or medical) model, and the behavioral model. Each of these models has very different practical implications about how patients are understood and treated. The shift from a psychodynamic or behavioral to a biological model will lead to very major changes in the clinical care of mental illness in the 1980s and 1990s. What are the practical implications of these three competing models? How do they affect the way doctors perceive their patients—and the way patients perceive their doctors? The differences between these three models are summarized in table 1.

The Psychodynamic Model

The *psychodynamic model* derives from the writings of Freud. Since Freud's time, however, many other psychoanalytic writers have added to or modified Freud's original ideas. These include such figures as his daughter, Anna Freud; Ernst Kris; Melanie Klein; Heinz Hartmann; Carl Jung; Erich Fromm; and Heinz Kohut, to mention only a few.

Table 1.
THREE MODELS OF MENTAL ILLNESS

	Psychodynamic	*Behavioral*	*Biological*
EMPHASIS	Mind	Behavior	Brain
CAUSES OF ILLNESS	Disturbed dynamics Childhood experiences	Learned habits	Biological imbalances
METHODS OF STUDY	Introspection (free association, dream analysis)	Controlled experiments (use of conditioning, animal research)	Neurosciences (neurochemistry, behavioral genetics)
TYPES OF ILLNESS	Mild (neuroses, personality disorders)	Mild to severe (neuroses, personality disorders, addictions)	Moderate to severe (depression, mania, schizophrenia)
METHOD OF TREATMENT	Psychotherapy	Behavior modification	Medication

Any summary of the work of so diverse a group of thinkers is inevitably an oversimplification. Nevertheless, several generalizations about the nature of the psychoanalytic model are probably true.

As mentioned earlier, although Freud began his medical career by studying the structure and workings of the brain (a physical part of the body), most of his life was devoted to studying the nature and workings of the *mind*. While the brain is something that can be seen, felt, and studied under a microscope, the mind is an abstract concept that usually refers to the activities the brain generates. Although Freud originally hoped that he would be able to relate his theories concerning the mind to scientific knowledge about the brain, he gradually abandoned this idea as his study of the mind consumed more and more of his time and effort.

Freud's early thinking was heavily influenced by the physics of his time, especially that of the Helmholtz School. He was imbued with this point of view during the five years he spent there as a medical student working with Ernst von Brücke, a Viennese neurophysiologist who founded a scientific movement known as the Helmholtz School of Medicine. One of the fundamental principles that influenced Freud's thinking was the notion of the conservation of energy promulgated by Mayer and Helmholtz. According to this theory, every isolated system has a constant amount of energy that can be discharged, and discharges in various parts of any system tend to remain in equilibrium or homeostasis. Freud applied these ideas to his thinking about the workings of the mind, which he wrote out in an essay during the

1890s, titled "Project for a Scientific Psychology," published only after his death. In Freud's thinking, the mind, like any other system, contained a certain amount of psychic energy. The human mind could be understood through examining the interplay of psychic forces striving to maintain an equilibrium. That is why Freudian psychology is called "psychodynamic."

From this physiological framework, Freud gradually developed a variety of theories that formed the foundation of classical psychoanalysis. While his contemporary neurologists, neuroanatomists, and psychiatrists were describing the structure of the brain, Freud described the structure of the psyche or mind. He divided psychic functions into three regions: the unconscious, the preconscious, and the conscious. The unconscious is characterized by primitive forms of thinking that Freud called "primary process thinking." This thinking is not directly available to consciousness and is expressed indirectly only through dreams or when censorship is relaxed during the process of free association. The unconscious is the repository of repressed ideas and unfulfilled wishes. According to Freud's thinking, much of the mental illness that he observed was due to an imbalance in the psychic equilibrium. Patients were using excessive amounts of psychic energy to keep primitive ideas under control, to ignore unfulfilled wishes that were unacceptable to their consciousnesses, and to repress unpleasant memories. When these unconscious drives were released and made conscious, a cure often occurred.

The unconscious could be made conscious in several different ways. Early in his career, Freud explored the use of hypnosis. Later, he discovered that when the patient relaxed on a couch and described without censorship any thoughts that came into his mind (the process of "free association"), this also led to the recovery of unconscious material. Using this approach and this foundation, Freud went on to evolve the psychoanalytic theories so familiar to many of us today, such as the Oedipus complex, the theory of infantile sexuality, and the division of the mind into id, ego, and superego.

The concern of this chapter is not to review the content of psychoanalytic theory, which is available from many different sources, but to examine its implications as a model for understanding mental illness and to compare it with two other major competing models, the behavioral model and the biological (or medical) model.

The psychodynamic model implies a certain set of assumptions about how mental illness should be approached, evaluated, and treated.

The subject matter explored by the psychodynamic model is the human mind (or psyche). The mind is an abstract or theoretical concept. Presumably, it ultimately represents the workings of the brain; but after Freud, psychodynamic thinkers made no effort to relate psychic function to brain function—they devoted their energies to defining a set of ideas that describe psychic functions. Their work has given us a group of terms and concepts that are widely used in both psychoanalysis and ordinary language: id, ego, superego; unconscious, preconscious, and conscious; primary and secondary process; libido, complex, drive, and dynamic conflict. These are terms and concepts that are useful descriptively and theoretically, but they have no known roots in physical reality.

As a scientific endeavor, its techniques involve the careful study of individual cases or a small series of similar cases in order to understand the mental mechanisms that lead to malfunction. Psychoanalytic research tends to be an intuitive and creative process. Following Freud's example, the psychoanalytic researcher is a careful observer who tries to understand what lies beneath the surface. He does not take things at face value and is in fact inclined to think that what seems most obvious is least likely to be true.

Its tools involve the use of introspection and the reporting of subjective experiences. In a clinical setting, the patient may free-associate, think aloud, or answer questions. Psychological tests of the type called "projective," such as the Rorschach (or "inkblot") test, may also be used as a vehicle to explore unconscious material, but the subject matter that is studied is always the verbal productions (or, in the case of children, play activity) of a human being.

The psychodynamic model tends to emphasize the study of milder mental illnesses and the enhancement of adaptive functioning in individuals who are essentially healthy. Sometimes these are referred to as "neuroses," "personality disorders," and "problems in daily living." When the model is applied narrowly, the ideal patient is an individual who is young, intelligent, and able to function reasonably well in everyday life, but who has a narrowly defined yet persistent psychological problem, such as difficulty in dealing with authority figures. More broadly defined, the psychodynamic model is used to treat patients with a wide variety of neuroses, such as difficulties with anxiety or mild depression, and more ingrained personality problems, such as difficulty in maintaining long-term relationships. The psychodynamic model has been applied to more-serious mental disorders, such as schizophrenia, but the results have not usually been very successful.

As a treatment technique, the psychodynamic model emphasizes the use of psychotherapy. When the model is applied narrowly, treatment sessions must occur several times a week. When it is applied more broadly, sessions can be less frequent, perhaps weekly or even every other week. Some psychodynamically oriented therapists see medication as inappropriate, since it may interfere with psychological treatment. Other psychodynamically oriented therapists are willing to prescribe medications occasionally.

Psychodynamic theories are not provable or testable to the same extent that other scientific theories may be. In their present form, they tend to be more philosophical than quantitative. Nevertheless, in developing psychoanalytic theory, Freud and his successors founded one major branch of the modern sciences of psychology and psychiatry. Psychodynamic theories have been used effectively to understand the workings of the human mind and to treat a variety of disorders, such as obsessions, compulsions, or anxiety. They continue to provide useful explanations of the origins of some neuroses, and insights concerning methods of treating them. During coming years, as more emphasis is placed on the medical orientation in psychiatry, psychoanalysts will probably begin to apply scientific methods and experimental designs to the study of psychodynamic principles. This approach will further strengthen the psychodynamic perspective.

The Behavioral Model

Behaviorism was launched by John B. Watson shortly after the introduction of Freud's ideas to this country. Followers of Watson presented their theories and research in reaction to the Freudian psychodynamic approach. Behaviorists such as Skinner, Wolpe, and Eysenck argue that the model used by Freud and his followers to understand the human mind is "unscientific"; only that which can be objectively observed and measured is allowed as evidence in understanding or treating mental illness. In contrast to the psychodynamic model, the tenets of the behavioral model are as follows:

The proper study of mankind is human behavior rather than the mind. Unlike psychodynamic theorists, behaviorists assume that the only things that are real (or at least worth studying) are the things we can see and observe. We cannot see the mind, the id, or the unconscious, but we can see how people act, react, and behave. From behavior we may be able to make inferences about the mind or brain, but they are not the primary focus of investigation. What people *do,* not what they *think* or *feel,* is the object of study. Likewise, the behaviorist does not look to the mind or brain to understand the causes of abnormal behavior. He assumes that such behavior represents learned habits, and he attempts to determine how they were learned.

As a scientific technique, the behavioral model emphasizes the use of carefully controlled experiments on animals and human beings. Experiments are defined in advance in order to explore a narrowly defined problem. For example, an investigator may choose to explore how frequently positive reinforcement must be given in order to maintain a behavior; thus, his experiment might compare rats pressing bars in Skinner boxes in order to obtain food pellets when the pellet is given each time the rat presses the bar *versus* every fifth time *versus* random reward as determined by the use of a random number table. In such an experiment, numerical data are generated that can be compared statistically. Little can be learned from the study of single cases. In order to permit measurement and quantification, reasonably large samples must be investigated.

The material that is studied is always behavior. Because behaviorists are not interested in the mind, or its more rarefied equivalents such as psyche or soul, inferences about the conditions that maintain and reinforce human behavior can be made from the study of animal behavior. While psychodynamic theories have occasionally attempted to use animal models, this approach has not been very fruitful. On the other hand, animal research has provided a very important foundation for the behavioral approach. Human behavior is, of course, another very important subject of study for the behaviorists. Like the psychodynamic investigator, the behaviorist is interested in understanding the mechanisms underlying the behavior of both normal individuals and those with problems that might be referred to as "mental illness."

When the behavioral model is applied to mental illness, it tends to be used for a wide variety of patients. It is perhaps most effective in treating behavioral disorders and disorders of impulse control, such as excessive drinking, obesity, or sexual problems. Behavioral approaches may also be quite useful in the treatment of anxiety and have occasionally been helpful in the management of more severe mental disorders such as schizophrenia. From the point of view of a behaviorist, the schizophrenic tends to withdraw and to hallucinate because he has learned that by behaving in this way he will either gain positive effects or avoid negative ones. Treatment consists simply of teaching this patient new behavior. Behavior therapists feel they can teach a schizophrenic patient to function more effectively in society by reinforcing normal behavior, such as participation in social activities, through giving rewards like access to cigarettes or good desserts, and by extinguishing abnormal behavior, such as social withdrawal, through giving the patient less appetizing meals or depriving him of cigarettes.

The primary methods of treatment involve teaching a patient new ways to modify his behavior. These are sometimes called "conditioning." One approach may involve negative conditioning, the techniques of which involve putting the patient in a situation that he wishes to learn to dislike and then training him to dislike it. For example, the alcoholic might be given liquor to drink and then be given an unpleasant stimulus, such as a drug that will make him vomit. After a series of such treatments, the patient no longer finds alcohol appealing. Unfortunately, the effects of negative conditioning tend to wear off rather quickly, and so this type of treatment is not used very often.

Positive reinforcement tends to be more effective. One common type, known as "reciprocal inhibition," is often used for phobias or anxiety. The patient is taught relaxation therapy—how to systematically and consistently relax various muscle groups in his body until he feels a pleasant state of total relaxation. After he has learned the techniques for relaxation, he is placed near the situation or stimulus that evokes his fear or anxiety and he is asked to assume the relaxed state of mind and body that he has learned to produce himself. Gradually he learns to gain control of the fear or anxiety through consciously relaxing himself in its presence. Behavior therapists, like the psychodynamically oriented therapists, tend to avoid the use of medication whenever possible, since they are concerned that it might interfere with the patient's ability to learn new behavioral controls.

Like psychodynamic theory, behaviorism has enriched our understanding of why people do the things they do and even how they think and feel. Narrowly applied, behaviorism can be arid and mechanistic. Like all potentially good things, it can be perverted to serve bad ends or used mindlessly and unimaginatively. Nevertheless, it provides a wholesome corrective to the sometimes ethereal theorizing of psychoanalysis. Its methods of treatment are helpful for some types of mental illnesses, such as alcoholism and other addictions.

The Biological Model

The biological model, sometimes referred to as the "medical model," derives from Kraepelin and other psychiatrists and neurologists of the late nineteenth and early twentieth centuries. In fact, however, its roots go back much farther. It represents the mainstream of medical traditions for understanding mental illness. From the time of the classical Greeks, mental illnesses have been assumed to be due to some type of aberration in body function. In classical times, when the theory of the four humors prevailed, mental illness was thought to be due to an imbalance in the body fluids. Depression (or melancholia), for example, was thought to be due to an excess of black bile.

In more recent times the biological model has been shaped by the growth of the discipline "neuroscience" or the neurosciences. Neuroscience is a combination of a set of related disciplines that share the common goal of understanding the relationship between brain structure and function, and human thoughts, feelings, and behavior. These disciplines include neuroanatomy (the study of brain structure), neuropathology (the study of disease processes caused by disorders of brain structure), neuropharmacology (the study of the effects of drugs on the brain), neurochemistry (the study of the chemical processes that control brain function), neuropsychology (the study of the relationship between various psychological or mental functions and brain structure), and neuroendocrinology (the study of the relationship between glandular function and brain function). Neurology and psychiatry are the two medical specialties that draw from and contribute to the neurosciences.

The boundaries between neurology and psychiatry are sometimes blurred. When these two specialties evolved in the nineteenth century, doctors tended to move freely between them, as Freud for example did. With increasing specialization, however, neurologists have tended to assume responsibility for diseases caused by precisely defined brain abnormalities, such as Parkinson's disease, or obvious large areas of injury, such as those caused by stroke or brain tumor. Usually these diseases are clinically manifested by such obvious signs as paralysis, shaking, or weakness. Psychiatry, on the other hand, has assumed responsibility for diseases that manifest themselves primarily by abnormalities in behavior, emotions, and thinking. Much of the time these abnormalities cannot be traced to a distinct area of damage in the brain, although the biological model assumes that as our knowledge progresses, some type of malfunction in the brain will be found. The current biological revolution in psychiatry places great emphasis on the search for the physical causes of mental illness.

The evolution of our understanding concerning a common neurological disorder, Parkinson's disease, helps us to understand both the problems and the purposes of the biologically oriented psychiatrist. Parkinson's disease was described by James Parkinson in 1817. It was called the "shaking palsy" because its victims suffered from a tendency to shake, especially noticeable in their hands, as well as a tendency to become stiff and rigid, sometimes so severe that they were nearly paralyzed. As techniques to study brain structure were developed, it was noted that victims of this disease had a loss of nerve cells in one particular quite small part of their brains. This area—called the "substantia nigra" because it is the only part of the brain that contains a dark pigment (*nigra* = black)—is located deep inside the brain and is considered a part of the group of brain structures governing body movement, the "motor system."

Neurochemistry then added another perspective. The neuroanatomist's discovery of atrophy in the substantia nigra suggested to the neurochemists that they should look in this area for possible neurochemical abnormalities. When they did, they noted that patients suffering from Parkinson's disease had a deficiency of a particular substance usually found in the substantia nigra, a chemical known as dopamine. Neuropharmacologists then suggested that a form of dopamine known as L-dopa could be given to people with Parkinson's disease to correct their chemical deficiency. The material was made available to neurologists, who began prescribing it for their patients approximately fifteen years ago. The availability of L-dopa has revolutionized the treatment of Parkinson's disease. Patients who receive L-dopa have a marked decrease in their troublesome symptoms, particularly rigidity. Many patients who were nearly incapacitated are now able to live nearly normal lives.

The case of Parkinson's disease illustrates that the neurosciences are indeed a group of related disciplines: They truly serve and interact with one another, and discoveries in one branch are often used by researchers or clinicians in another branch. Further, while a neuroscientist may work within a particular discipline, such as neurology or neurochemistry, he must be aware of developments in all the other neurosciences because their interactions are so close. As this book will explain in subsequent chapters, modern psychiatry is progressing rapidly toward discovering the anatomic and biochemical abnormalities that underlie mental illnesses and toward developing pharmacological methods for treating them. Although none of the mental illnesses is as yet as fully understood as Parkinson's disease, biologically oriented psychiatrists hope that during the next ten to twenty years a similar logical progression from understanding structure to understanding cause to developing treatment will unfold for major mental illnesses such as depression or schizophrenia. The modern biologically oriented psychiatrist is truly the descendant of Emil Kraepelin, whose Department of Psychiatry in Munich was composed of clinicians, neuroanatomists, and neuropathologists. What are the tenets of the biological model, and how will it affect the treatment of mental illness during the 1980s?

The major psychiatric illnesses are diseases. They should be considered medical illnesses just as diabetes, heart disease, and cancer are. The emphasis in this model is on carefully diagnosing each specific illness from which the patient suffers, just as an internist or neurologist would. When an internist listens to a patient complain of shortness of breath, he immediately begins to think of a "differential diagnosis," enumerating in his mind the various diseases that might cause the patient's complaint. The psychiatrist who follows the biological model works in the same way. When a patient complains of such symptoms as low energy, insomnia, or hearing voices, the psychiatrist assumes that the patient has a specific illness and proceeds through a detailed history and physical examination in order to determine what type of illness the patient has.

These diseases are caused principally by biological factors, and most of these factors reside in the brain. The brain is the organ of the body that serves to monitor and control the rest of the bodily functions, as well as providing the source and storehouse of all psychological functions, such as thoughts, memories, feelings, interests, and personality.

As a scientific discipline, psychiatry seeks to identify the biological factors that cause mental illness. This search involves all aspects of the neurosciences. As remaining chapters in this book will show, a large amount of evidence has been amassed suggesting that mental illness is caused by biochemical abnormalities, neuroendocrine abnormalities, structural brain abnormalities, and genetic abnormalities.

Clinical evaluation of patients involves careful history-taking, observing the course of symptoms over time, physical examination, and sometimes laboratory tests. This model assumes that each different type of illness has a different specific cause. Therefore, making the correct diagnosis is very important. The understanding of each specific disease, the search for its cause, and the decision about appropriate treatment is aided by carefully observing the symptoms of the illness, its course over time, and the extent to which other members of the patient's family have had similar problems.

The biological model tends to emphasize the study and management of more serious or severe mental illnesses. These include depression, inappropriate elevations of mood (or mania), schizophrenia, severe anxiety disorders, and illnesses leading to senility (or the dementias). These diseases are emphasized because they are the ones thought most likely to have biological causes.

The treatment of these diseases emphasizes the use of "somatic therapies." The term *somatic therapies* refers to a diverse group of treatments whose common feature is that they are all physical in nature. The somatic therapies used most frequently are medications and electroconvulsive therapy (ECT). Because these diseases are considered to be biological in origin, the therapy is seen as correcting an underlying biological imbalance. Nevertheless, like any good physician, a biologically oriented psychiatrist also recognizes that mental illness may affect social and economic functioning and addresses his attention to these problems as well. For example, a patient who is depressed and has no sex drive may develop marital problems. Ideally, the biologically oriented psychiatrist will recognize that he is treating the whole patient and that his emphasis should include helping the patient with all aspects of his or her life.

The return of many psychiatrists to the biological model is likely to dramatically change the nature of health care in the 1980s. Patients who go to a psychiatrist expecting to talk with him for a "fifty-minute hour" at each visit will be surprised to discover that visits are sometimes much shorter. Rather than free-associating, the patient will be asked a series of detailed questions about his symptoms, his family history of illness, and his general medical history. The psychiatrist may not even ask what the patient thinks about his mother or about traumatic early life experiences. Instead, after spending an hour or two taking a careful history of the patient's symptoms, the doctor may pull out a prescription pad, briefly explain his diagnosis and the reason for the prescription, outline the side effects and dose regimen of the drug, and ask the patient to come back in one or two weeks. When the patient returns, the doctor may spend only fifteen to thirty minutes determining whether or not the patient is getting better and how his symptoms have been affecting his work and his family and social life.

Patients who expect a psychiatrist to spend considerable amounts of time listening or talking often feel hurt or neglected when they see a biologically oriented psychiatrist, at least until they realize that the biological approach is quite different from the psychodynamic one that they are accustomed to equating with psychiatry. On the other hand, once they become accustomed to it, many patients feel quite comfortable with the biological model. It also carries implications about the nature of mental illness that may be very beneficial.

Mental illnesses are not due to "bad habits" or weakness of will. Because they are illnesses, they cannot be cured by acts of will. Many patients suffering from illnesses such as severe depression or mania feel guilty about their symptoms and responsible for experiencing them. Their guilt only makes them feel worse. When patients realize that their illnesses are probably caused by chemical or other types of physical abnormalities, they are relieved of feeling guilty. They no longer see themselves as inherently bad or worthless because they have a mental illness.

Mental illnesses are not caused by bad parenting or bad "spousing." Just as the patient is relieved from guilt about his symptoms, so are his friends and relatives. The parent of a child with depression or schizophrenia no longer needs to agonize over what he or she did wrong. The husband or wife of a patient suffering from depression no longer needs to feel that he or she brought on the illness by being too demanding, or not demanding enough.

The somatic therapies are very effective methods for treating many mental illnesses. As biological psychiatry has progressed during the past twenty years, various specific kinds of medication have been developed to treat the different specific illnesses that have been recognized. Many of these medications are almost miraculously effective. The patient complaining of insomnia, low mood, and loss of appetite (usually feeling miserable and hopeless and convinced that his symptoms can never be cured) is frequently astonished to find that antidepressant medication relieves the symptoms almost completely within several weeks.

Not all biological treatments are miraculous cures, of course, and it is important that neither doctor nor patient has excessively high expectations. Most medical illnesses can be ameliorated by medication, but very few are eradicated by medication. Penicillin is truly a "miracle drug" that destroys the bacteria causing pneumonia, but except for infectious diseases and a few diseases that are treated surgically, most of the illnesses that afflict human beings are improved by doctors but not cured by them. Aspirin relieves the pain of arthritis, and nitroglycerine relieves the pain of angina. Antidepressant medications are somewhat closer to providing a "cure" for depression than either aspirin for arthritis or nitroglycerine for angina, but it is important not to expect too much. Psychiatry in the past has tended to oversell what it is able to do for people. Biological psychiatry promises some help, and often a great deal of help, but it does not guarantee a miraculous cure for every patient.

The remainder of this book explains in more detail the recent discoveries and contributions of biological psychiatry, which will revolutionize the treatment of mental illness during the 1980s and 1990s. It is a road map that will give people accurate information about the recent explosion of knowledge in the neurosciences in general and psychiatry in particular. This information will be helpful to those who want to find out more about biologically oriented methods for understanding and treating mental illness. Most of this information is not widely available to the general public, because it involves technical research described in scientific and medical journals. This book attempts to state the results of that research in simple, clear, nontechnical language. Using this knowledge, people who want accurate and up-to-date information about the most modern developments in psychiatry may be spared searching down blind alleys, following dead-end streets, or wandering lost on secondary roads.

4

WHAT IS MENTAL ILLNESS?:

Four Major Syndromes

O the mind, mind has mountains, cliffs of fall
Frightful, sheer, no-man-fathomed. Hold them cheap
May who ne'er hung there.

—GERARD MANLEY HOPKINS

As the philosopher Ludwig Wittgenstein has pointed out, people have a tendency to assume that when there is only one word or term used to refer to a thing, there is also only one thing. In the case of "mental illness," Wittgenstein's observation provides a very useful insight. Most people who think about the subject of mental illness spend too much time asking the question that forms the title to this chapter, which is essentially a philosophical question rather than a medical one. Although a number of people have tried, to date no one has managed to develop successful, logical, and nontautological definitions of medical concepts such as disease, health, physical illness, or mental illness. When a question leads to much heat and little light, as has the question "What is mental illness," one begins to sense that one is traveling through the realms of philosophy—and may remain lost there forever like a lotus-eater if she does not have a firm sense of both direction and goal.

On the other hand, if one modifies the question to make it practical rather than philosophical, answers come trippingly off the tongue. If one asks "What are the common mental illnesses?" there is astonishing agreement. Most physicians who treat the mentally ill would come up with similar lists: schizophrenia, affective disorders, and anxiety disorders, for example. (In similar fashion, a pediatrician could quickly list measles, mumps, and chicken pox as common childhood illnesses even though she could not define *childhood illness.*) Mental illness is an abstract concept, with disputable defining characteristics and debatable boundaries. On the other hand, the mental illnesses are well-recognized disorders with typical characteristics. There are many different types of mental illness, just as there are many different pediatric diseases, and they differ (sometimes greatly) in their severity, symptoms, outcome, and effect on the patient's life. That is why it is difficult to come up with a single definition that will include and accurately describe all of them. Lay people are often confused by the idea of mental illness because they think of it as a single thing, while at the same time their actual life experiences tell them that people receiving psychiatric treatment are very different from one another. That is, of course, due in part to differences in personality among individual patients, but it is also often due to the fact that they are suffering from different diseases.

This chapter contains a description of the four most common types of relatively severe mental illness treated by psychiatrists: affective disorders, schizophrenia, anxiety disorders, and dementias. While other disorders are also recognized by psychiatrists, these four are clearly the most important of those mental illnesses that are considered to have some biological cause. They are the most important because they affect a large number of people and cause a relatively severe degree of suffering. In Hopkins's words, they are "cliffs of fall frightful," and unfortunately many have hung there.

The descriptions contained in this chapter present much of the same information that might be found in any psychiatric textbook. They should give the average person a good sense of what mental illnesses are like, both from the perspective of the patient and from the perspective of the psychiatrist. As you read the following descriptions, you will notice recurring themes that you should keep in mind, for these themes form the defining features of a specific illness, or what doctors like to refer to as a "syndrome" (a group of characteristics that tend to occur together). How common is it? What are its characteristic symptoms? What happens to these symptoms over the course of weeks, months, or years? (Do they get better or worse? Are they episodic or chronic?) How much does the illness affect the person's ability to work, to have a normal family life and social life, to think clearly and have well-tuned emotional responses? How well does the illness respond to the treatments currently available?

Affective Disorders

The affective disorders are the most common psychiatric disorders. They include two main groups of illnesses: bipolar or manic disorders and depressive disorders. At any given time, 4 people out of 100 are suffering from a relatively severe depressive syndrome. Approximately 10 people out of 100 will experience a significant depression at some time in their lives, and recent evidence indicates that the rate may be even higher than that, perhaps even as high as 20 percent. Manic disorder, characterized by grandiosity and poor judgment that may alternate with depression, is relatively rare and affects only .5 to 1 percent of the population.

As their name indicates, the affective disorders are characterized primarily by a disturbance in affect or mood. In psychiatry the word *affect* refers to the emotional coloring and responsivity with which people view the world. Normal affect is said to be "neutral," but it also responds to pleasant events with happiness and to unpleasant events with sadness, and such responsivity is considered appropriate as long as it does not swing into uncontrolled extremes. In the affective disorders, such uncontrolled extremes occur either in the form of excessive elation or excessive unhappiness, and the two clinical syndromes associated with these extremes are referred to as "mania" and "depression." Most patients suffering from affective disorder experience some form of depression, but those who experience mood swings between the two "poles" of affective disorder are referred to as "bipolar."

The existence of affective disorders has been recognized for thousands of years, and they have been well described in both medicine and literature. Medical texts from Pharaonic Egypt indicate that the depressive syndrome was recognized at least 3,000 years ago. The description in 1 Samuel of Saul's terrible melancholy, written in the eighth century B.C., is perhaps the oldest detailed case history. Saul, subject to severe episodes of despondency, became incapacitated, guilt-ridden, and hopeless. At first he responded to the therapy of

David's soothing music, but later he became so severely depressed that he lost touch with reality and became psychotic. While apparently insane, he tried to kill David and his own son, Jonathan, as well as summoning up the spirit of Samuel through the medium of the "Witch of Endor." Melancholia and mania were thoroughly described by Hippocratic medical texts in classical times. Many great historical figures in a variety of fields have also suffered affective syndromes, including Oliver Cromwell, Samuel Johnson, Abraham Lincoln, Robert Schumann, Martin Luther, John Keats, Vincent van Gogh, Robert Lowell, Sylvia Plath, and Ernest Hemingway.

Because they are so common, the affective disorders touch the lives of nearly all of us. The recent novel and movie *Ordinary People* has poignantly and accurately portrayed how a young teen-ager may struggle with depressive symptoms, benefit from electroconvulsive therapy, and feel belittled by the stigma of having suffered mental illness. It also portrays how the relatives of a person suffering from depression may struggle with their own feelings and sense of responsibility, and how failure to understand and work through these feelings can destroy a once strong family relationship.

THE NATURE OF DEPRESSIVE DISORDERS

The following is a relatively typical case history of a patient with depressive disorder. Like all the case histories in this chapter, it is based on an actual case, with names and details of the history changed so that the particular patient cannot be recognized.

> Mary Williams is a fifty-six-year-old married woman who is employed as a secretary. She went to see her family doctor complaining of insomnia, poor appetite, and weight loss. He recognized that she was suffering from a depressive syndrome and referred her to a psychiatrist for further treatment.
>
> Her symptoms had begun approximately three months earlier when she fell and fractured her wrist. The injury was not serious, but she had to have her hand in a cast and was unable to work for several months. She found this rather distressing, since she had been employed as an executive secretary at IBM for nearly fifteen years and was convinced that her employer would have trouble getting along without her. She also did not know what to do with herself during the long days at home.

Shortly after the injury, she began to have trouble sleeping. She would awaken at 3:00 or 4:00 in the morning and would lie awake for the next four or five hours thinking about things that she had done wrong in the past. She became particularly preoccupied with the fact that she had occasionally taken office supplies home, such as paper and envelopes, for her own personal use. She felt she should confess this to her employer, and perhaps even to her minister. Her husband tried to reassure her that her boss would not really care, but she could not be persuaded. Her appetite diminished and she lost approximately ten pounds over two and a half months. Finally, she sought out her boss and, with great anxiety, explained that she had to tell him about something terrible she had done at the office. When he learned that her serious offense was limited to using a few packages of paper and envelopes over the course of fifteen years, he assured her that he knew employees did this from time to time, and that he did not consider it a major offense unless it was excessive. He did express concern that she seemed so nervous and upset and suggested that she should perhaps see a doctor. In spite of his comforting and under-standing response, she continued to worry about her "sin." She began to tell her husband and children that she was a worthless and evil person and that they would be much better off without her.

She also began to lose interest in all her favorite recreational activities, which included sewing for her grandchildren and reading spy stories. When her daughter told her that she was expecting a new grandchild in seven months, Mary (who doted on her grandchildren) responded in a surprising way: She shook her head disapprovingly and commented that it is wrong to bring any more children into the world, since it is such an evil place.

In the week before she went to see her family doctor, she became increasingly anxious and restless, pacing around and unable to sit still. Her feelings of guilt increased, and she began to talk about calling the police to tell them about her "crimes." When her family asked her what she had done that was so terribly wrong, she replied vaguely that it was too terrible to discuss with "decent people." She wished that the police would just come and arrest her so that she could be tried and sentenced. She also began to talk more and more about how everyone would be better off without her. She was taken to see her family doctor and later a psychiatrist.

When the psychiatrist evaluated her, he observed a plump, gray-haired woman whose face had an expression of misery and anguish.

She described herself as feeling extremely sad, anxious, and pessimistic. She burst into tears several times as she described her "sin" of stealing office supplies. She described herself as overwhelmed with feelings of guilt, worthlessness, and hopelessness. She twisted her hands almost continuously and played nervously with her hair. She stated that her family would be better off without her and that she had considered taking her life by hanging herself. She felt that after death she would go to hell, where she would experience eternal torment, but that this would be a just punishment for her "sin."

Ten years prior to this illness, the patient had had a similar episode, which her family described as "virtually identical." She was hospitalized at that time, treated with antidepressant medication, and responded well. Both the patient and her family agreed that she recovered fully and returned to her usual self, with no signs of mental illness during the intervening years.

The patient grew up in a large, middle-class Catholic family. Her father was a policeman who was steadily promoted to higher administrative posts during the course of his career. She described her childhood home life as strict, but also warm and affectionate. She was an outgoing, sociable girl and an above-average student. After graduating from high school, she took a secretarial course and worked for several years. She was married at age twenty to an insurance salesman, had several children, but returned to work to supplement the family income and to keep herself busy after the children entered grade school. Her husband and children described her as conscientious, efficient, and generally good-humored. They described her two episodes of depression as something "quite different" from her usual self.

This patient was treated with tricyclic antidepressant medication. She improved markedly within three weeks and returned home to resume her usual routine. (Possible risks of various kinds of treatment will be discussed in more detail in chapter 8.)

This case history illustrates many common features of the depressive syndrome. The outlook for patients suffering from depression is usually quite good. Most depressions respond well to medication, and the few that do not respond usually remit after electroconvulsive therapy. On the other hand, depressions tend to recur. The patient is typically well for many months or many years, but approximately 30–50 percent of patients who have had a depression at one time are likely to have another at some later time in their lives. Sylvia Plath described her own experience with depression as like being inside a bell jar, a suffocating and destructive force that separates one from life and distorts one's perception of it; and she described her fear of recurrence as a dread that the bell jar might descend to suffocate her again. Depression is psychologically very painful to those who experience it, and its pain is not easily forgotten. The fear of suffering another depression tends to haunt people, even when they have responded well to medication in the past and recognize that they are likely to do so again.

We do not fully understand how depressions are triggered. Sometimes they have obvious precipitants, as was the case with Conrad Jarrett in *Ordinary People,* who became depressed when his brother, Buck, died in a boating accident that he survived. Other depressions appear to come out of the blue, as did Sylvia Plath's first episode, which began after her sophomore year at Smith while she was in New York on a coveted *Mademoiselle* guest editorship. Some patients have clear precipitants for some episodes, but not for others, as was the case with Bill, whose depressive illness was described in chapter 1. Sometimes depressions begin after a physical stress, as occurred in the case history above, but sometimes they begin when the patient has not experienced any kind of unusual event. Such patients say, "I just don't understand it. There is no reason for me to feel this way." In earlier days, depressions that began without any obvious outside stress were said to be "endogenous" (or to grow from within); this type of depression was thought to be more biologically based, more severe, and more likely to respond to somatic therapy. Depressions occurring after a stress were called "reactive" and considered to be purely psychological. More-recent research suggests that this view is an oversimplification. Various kinds of psychological stress, such as a death in the family or even a happy event such as winning an award, may initiate a physical response in the body that may eventually trigger depressive symptoms.

Because all of us have experienced various kinds of personal loss and unhappiness, nearly everyone has experienced a disturbance in mood at some time in his or her life. Since the syndrome has been frequently described in magazines, Sunday supplements, and paperbacks, many people have become familiar with its characteristic symptomatology. Some people may even read descriptions of the depressive syndrome and arrive at a psychiatrist's office with a self-made diagnosis of depression, detailing the symptoms garnered from the Sunday supplement, and request lithium or one of the magical antidepressants. A few of these people may indeed have a full depressive syndrome, but others are only transiently unhappy.

Psychiatrists do not always agree with one another on how and where the line demarcating depression from unhappiness should be drawn. Those psychiatrists who have a more biological orientation prefer to restrict the use of the term *depression* to more severe forms that are likely to respond to medication. Those who operate from a medical model see the disorder as a disease that is physically based, and do not include within the depressive syndromes those patients who are simply experiencing a short-lived sorrow that will pass within hours or days. The medically oriented psychiatrist operationalizes his narrow definition by restricting it to patients who have had a substantial number of depressive symptoms for a minimum period of time (usually two to four weeks) in order to exclude patients with a milder, transient syndrome. Psychiatrists who have a more psychodynamic orientation tend to use the term more broadly, so that some may observe depression in a majority of the patients they see.

Depression is marked by a characteristic set of symptoms. The basic abnormality in depression is an alteration in mood or affect: A person who is depressed feels sad, despondent, "down in the dumps," blue, and full of despair and hopelessness. This is often referred to as "dysphoric mood" (*dys* = bad, painful; *phoric* = bear, carry). Occasionally patients with depression will complain of feeling anxious or tense rather than sad or despondent. More rarely, a patient who is seriously depressed does not recognize his dysphoric mood, although he might seem sad or anxious to an outside observer; instead, he complains bitterly of some physical symptom that is bothering him or of his inability to sleep.

In addition to the alteration in mood, the depressive syndrome is usually accompanied by a group of symptoms that are sometimes referred to as "vegetative" (because they involve basic biological functions), such as insomnia or decreased appetite. These vegetative symptoms are the hallmark of a severe and biologically based depression. Insomnia may take one of several forms: Some patients may have trouble falling asleep; others wake up in the middle of the night and sleep fitfully; yet others awaken early in the morning and are unable to return to sleep. Most people with insomnia worry and ruminate during the time when they are lying awake. People who have the type of insomnia with early-morning awakening tend to have more severe forms of depression. The following sonnet by Gerard Manley Hopkins provides a very moving personal account of how the insomnia of the depressed person feels subjectively.

> I wake and feel the fell of dark, not day.
> What hours, O what black hours we have spent
> This night! what sights you, heart, saw; ways you went!
> And more must, in yet longer light's delay.
>   With witness I speak this. But where I say
> Hours I mean years, mean life. And my lament
> Is cries countless, cries like dead letters sent
> To dearest him that lives alas! away.
>   I am gall, I am heartburn. God's most deep decree
> Bitter would have me taste: my taste was me;
> Bones built in me, flesh filled, blood brimmed the curse.
>   Selfyeast of spirit a dull dough sours. I see
> The lost are like this, and their scourge to be
> As I am mine, their sweating selves; but worse.

While insomnia is the most typical disturbance, some people who are depressed complain of a need to sleep excessively. They feel chronically tired and spend ten to fourteen hours a day in bed.

A person with depression usually complains of decreased appetite and may lose weight. Sometimes a depressed person will force herself to eat in spite of decreased appetite, or she may be urged or encouraged by a parent or spouse, so that the weight loss is minimal. Less frequently, depression expresses itself as a desire to eat excessively and is accompanied by weight gain. A depressive syndrome characterized by either excessive sleep or excessive appetite may tend to be more chronic and less likely to respond to somatic therapy.

"Diurnal variation," another vegetative symptom, is a fluctuation of mood during the course of a twenty-four-hour day. Most typically, the patient states that her mood is worse in the morning, but that it improves slightly as the day progresses, so that she feels best in the evening. Less frequently, the pattern is reversed, with the patient stating that she feels best in the morning. This fluctuation in mood related to the time of day may reflect an underlying disturbance in the endocrine functions that regulate our level of alertness throughout the day. Sometimes people with depression also experience a marked decrease in sex drive so that they have no interest in sex or have trouble achieving orgasm or obtaining an erection. The depressed patient may also complain of constipation or dry mouth. This clustering of vegetative symptoms in depression has led many investigators to hypothesize an underlying disruption of the monitoring of bodily functions by the brain.

The generalized slowing and sadness of depression is also expressed in a variety of emotional symptoms. Patients lose interest in activities that they have enjoyed previously, such as sports, traveling, or reading. They may withdraw socially and avoid seeing old friends or making new ones. They are unable to experience joy or pleasure even when something particularly pleasant occurs, such as being paid a compliment or achieving some important goal. They often feel that their energy is markedly decreased so that they are no longer able to do as many things as they used to. A depressed person frequently complains of difficulty in concentrating, or is unable to follow a football game or a story. The depressed person may lose confidence in himself so that he is fearful of going to work, taking examinations, or assuming responsibility for household tasks. He may avoid answering the phone or returning phone calls in order to avoid the responsibilities of social relationships he feels unable to handle. He may become completely hopeless and full of despair, believing that his situation can never be improved, or even that he does not deserve to feel better. The depressed person may feel quite guilty over actual or fantasied misdeeds that he has committed in the past. Usually the "misdeed" is seen as more terrible than it actually was, so that the person believes he will be condemned to hell forever for masturbating as a child or sent to prison for life for taking a questionable deduction on his income-tax return. Some patients become preoccupied with death and begin to consider suicide.

Patients who are severely depressed may experience psychotic symptoms such as delusions or hallucinations. These are usually consistent with the depressed mood, which makes them different from the delusions and hallucinations of the schizophrenias. For example, the depressed person may hear the voice of God or of the devil telling him that he has fallen so far from God's ways that his soul is lost forever. He may begin to believe that the world is coming to an end and to think that he has received various "signs" as indicators of its impending demise. He may develop the delusion that the FBI or police are following him and bugging his house or office to catch him in the various misdeeds that his pathological guilt makes him believe he has committed. He may begin to think that he has a fatal disease that is consuming his body and making his internal organs rot away. All these mistaken ideas are consistent with feeling sad or depressed. Consequently, psychiatrists refer to them as "mood-congruent."

Although the delusions and hallucinations may seem so striking that they appear to be the most salient feature of the disorder, it is important to realize that even in these "psychotic depressions" the basic disturbance is one of mood and that these symptoms will disappear when the mood returns to normal. Patients with psychotic depression are not losing their minds and are not likely to remain abnormal for the rest of their lives. Psychotic depressions usually respond quite well to somatic therapies.

Patients who are depressed may also experience symptoms referred to as "psychomotor agitation" or "psychomotor retardation." The retarded patient may sit quietly in a chair for hours without speaking to anyone, simply staring into space. When he gets up and moves about, he walks slowly, his speech is slowed, and his replies are laconic. If asked about his thinking, he may complain that it is markedly slowed down. On the other hand, the agitated patient is restless and seems extremely nervous. She may complain more of anxiety than depression. She is unable to sit in a chair and frequently paces about. She may wring her hands or perform other stereotyped and repetitive nervous gestures, such as drumming her fingers on a table, pulling at her hair or clothing, or playing with objects in her hands. Her speech is usually somewhat rapid, and she may complain in a high-pitched, staccato whine of the various miseries that she is suffering.

Occasionally patients experience "masked depression." This term means that the patient does not complain of dysphoric mood or appear to have a full set of depressive symptoms, but is nevertheless depressed. For example, an older person may complain to his doctor of physical symptoms such as headache or dizziness that make him unable to concentrate, to work, or to sleep. He will deny that his mood is despondent or anxious, saying that he is indeed upset but would feel fine if only the physical symptoms were corrected. Although a careful medical work-up reveals no abnormalities, the patient usually continues to insist on the importance of the physical symptoms. If these patients are treated with antidepressant medication, their "masked depression" often clears, and the cluster of physical complaints tends to disappear or diminish significantly.

Suicide is the most serious complication of depression. Approximately 15 percent of all hospitalized patients suffering from depression die by suicide eventually. Several factors are suggestive of an increase in suicidal risk: being divorced or living alone; history of alcohol or drug abuse; age over forty; a history of a previous suicide attempt; or an expression of suicidal thoughts (especially when detailed plans have been formulated). Patients who appear to have a suicidal intent should be treated in a hospital.

Although suicide is the most serious complication of depression, other social and personal complications may also occur. Decreased energy, poor concentration, and lack of interest may cause poor performance at school or at work. Apathy and decreased sexual interest may lead to marital discord. Patients may attempt to treat depressive symptoms themselves with sedatives, alcohol, or stimulants, thereby starting problems with drug and alcohol abuse.

THE NATURE OF MANIC DISORDERS

While it is not always easy to distinguish biologically based depression from simple unhappiness, the distinction between manic disorder and normality is usually much easier—at least for everyone except the patient himself. The person with manic disorder is pathologically happy. It is hard to say someone "suffers" from manic disorder, because the patient usually enjoys feeling the way he does. He tends to have boundless energy, enthusiasm, and superficial goodwill. Many manics refuse to admit that they have any problems, and they may resist treatment because their sense of psychological well-being is so great. Indeed, the manic state would be ideal if it were not accompanied by other, less fortunate symptoms, such as irritability and poor judgment. The following case history describes a typical manic episode occurring in a young person.

Mike Willard is a twenty-year-old college student. He was brought to the hospital by the police because of complaints by his neighbors that he had been noisy and disruptive. When asked about his problems, he replied: "I feel great. It's my girlfriend who has a problem."

Information collected from the patient, his family, and his friends over the next several days indicated that he had been perfectly normal until about six weeks earlier. He had been a B+ student and was described by his friends and parents as being friendly, hardworking, but at times a bit moody. Approximately six weeks before he was brought to the emergency room by the police, he broke up with a girlfriend whom he had been dating steadily for the previous year. During the next several weeks he became tense, irritable, and had difficulty sleeping. He also became distractible, complained of difficulty in concentrating, and began to have trouble completing his schoolwork. He had two term papers assigned, for which he would go to the library and accumulate hundreds of bibliography cards on a variety of possible topics. Unable to decide on a specific subject and changing his ideas almost daily, he began to accumulate large stacks of 3 × 5 cards in his room. He impulsively purchased an $800 classical guitar, although he had no knowledge of how to play it and was in fact unable to read music. When he thought some money was missing from his room, he assumed that one of his friends had "borrowed it without asking," accused the friend, and beat him up when he denied it. When he later realized that he had simply misplaced the money, he refused to apologize to his friend, stating that it was a natural mistake to have made.

As his need for sleep decreased further, he stayed up all night playing music, looking through his bibliography cards, phoning friends long-distance, and formulating plans to write a definitive work on "existentialism, Divine Providence, and the collective unconscious." He felt ideas were coming to him so quickly that he could scarcely write them down. His room was soon filled with sheets of paper that had a sentence or two written on them. He often called friends in the middle of the night to read them something he had just written or to relate some insight that he had just received. Most of his insights were clichés that made no sense at all. For example, he called one friend to explain that "the world is like an orange." There was no indication that he was using any illicit drugs during this time that might account for his unusual behavior.

He was admitted to the hospital when he decided to attempt a reconciliation with his girlfriend, went to her house at 2:00 A.M., and began tearing off his clothes, shouting, and pounding on the door when she refused to see him. Some neighbor phoned the police, who brought him to the hospital after picking him up, because of his peculiar behavior and incoherent speech.

When he arrived at the emergency room, the patient had a somewhat disheveled appearance, with a stubbly beard and reddened eyes. He was dressed casually in a T-shirt, cutoff jeans, and running shoes. His mood shifted rapidly from euphoria to irritation as he explained his plans to write a definitive book on existentialism and psychology, and then complained about the police disturbing him. He talked very rapidly, often leaving sentences incomplete, and shifted abruptly from one idea to another so that much of the time his speech made little sense. He was unable to answer questions in adequate detail, always shifting the subject back to himself, his special plans, and his special mission in life. He moved restlessly in his chair and frequently stood up and walked around the room. Several times he angrily requested that he be allowed to return to his apartment, since he had so much important work to do. He denied experiencing hallucinations or any sense of interference with his thoughts, although he wondered if he might not be able to influence others through his own "mind karma."

Mike had had a remarkably normal childhood and adolescence. He was a good student, a good athlete, and participated in many extracurricular activities in high school. He started university two years ago and continued to do well. Other members of his family had had mental illness, however. His mother had been treated for depression with medications four years previously and responded well after several months. A maternal uncle had numerous hospitalizations for both mania and depression.

Mike was treated with lithium. He responded within two weeks and was able to leave the hospital, although he remained on a maintenance dose of lithium. Later he experienced relatively severe depressive symptoms. At this time he was put on tricyclic antidepressant medication. His depressive symptoms responded after one month, and he did not require rehospitalization.

This young man has relatively typical bipolar affective disorder. As is often the case, an episode of mania was followed rather closely by an episode of depression. Lithium treatment is sometimes successful in preventing depressive relapses, but it did not work well in this particular case. Episodes of mania usually respond to treatment within a few days to a few weeks. They tend to be briefer and to have a more abrupt termination than depressive episodes. The outlook for any particular episode is good, especially with the availability of effective treatments such as lithium, but the risk of recurrence is significant.

As in depression, the basic abnormality in mania is an alteration in mood, so that the person feels happier than usual, irritable, grandiose, or expansive. In contrast to the dysphoric mood of depression, the mood of manic patients is often characterized as "euphoric" (*eu* = good, well). This change in mood is accompanied by other symptoms of mania, such as increased activity, decreased need for sleep, poor judgment, pressured or distractible speech, and inflated self-esteem. Typically, the manic patient's mood is cheerful and enthusiastic. Since the euphoric mood is subjectively pleasant to experience, the patient may deny that he has any problems, reporting instead, "I feel great! Better than ever!" The change in mood may be apparent only to friends or relatives familiar with the patient's usual and customary behavior.

Since experiencing a "good mood" is desirable, it may be hard to tell mild euphoria, characteristic of an early manic syndrome, from normal happiness. But the presence of other typical manic symptoms, such as poor judgment or decreased need for sleep, provides the clues that the person has some type of mental illness. While most manic patients are quite happy, some may experience only irritability. Such patients become short-tempered, aggressive in defending their ideas, sometimes verbally or physically abusive, and difficult to live with, particularly when their goals or plans are thwarted.

A person "suffering" from mania is usually more active than usual. Projects or business ventures are typically begun on impulse, with poor planning, and rarely carried to completion. The person may become more interested in sex than usual, exhausting his mate's appetite or energy, making inappropriate overtures to strangers or to casual acquaintances, or becoming involved in an extramarital affair when previously faithful. He may become more social and gregarious, going to bars, planning parties, or calling friends at all hours of the night. The increased energy and interest are typically accompanied by a decreased need for sleep. The patient often awakens several hours early and may go for days on end with very little sleep at all. Unlike the depressive, the manic feels fresh and rested when he awakens early and typically bounds out of bed ready to get on with the day's activities.

Sometimes friends and relatives notice changes in the way the person talks that may be the first obvious symptom of illness. The person becomes excessively talkative and sometimes does not seem to make sense. The speech of manics is often rapid, loud, and difficult to interpret. Sentences are left uncompleted because of eagerness to get on to a new idea. A simple question that could be answered in only a few words is answered at great length with great enthusiasm and garrulousness. A reply takes minutes rather than seconds, and some manics will talk for an hour without stopping if not interrupted. Even when interrupted, the manic often continues to talk, shouting to drown out the other person. Psychiatrists call this speech pattern in mania "pressure of speech." Sometimes manics with severe "pressured speech" will talk without any social stimulation and will talk even though no one is listening. When manic patients are given medications such as lithium or phenothiazines, their speech may be slowed by the medication, but it still may not make much sense. This is because manics tend to think very rapidly but to leave their thoughts unfinished, a symptom psychiatrists refer to as "flight of ideas." Manics also tend to be quite distractible. Thus they jump from one subject to another when they talk, and the changes may be so abrupt that the person is hard to understand.

The following is an example of this type of manic speech. The patient is replying to the question "Tell me what you're like." This is only a brief excerpt taken from the beginning of his response, which continued without interruption for a half-hour. The patient is a senior partner in a prominent law firm, and a man with prestigious political connections. The example illustrates how the speech of highly articulate people can deteriorate during a manic episode.

Ah, one hell of an odd thing to say perhaps in these particular circumstances, I happen to be quite pleased with who I am or how I am and many of the problems that I have and have been working on I have are difficult for me to handle or to work on because I am not aware of them as problems which upset me personally. I have to get my feelers way out to see how it is and where that what may be or seem to be is distressing, too painful or uncomfortable to people who make a difference to me emotionally and personally or possibly on an economic or professional level. And I am I think becoming more aware that perhaps on an analogy the matter of some who understand or enjoy loud rages and anger, the same thing can be true for other people, and I have to kind of try to learn to see when that's true and what I can do about it.

Disorganized thinking and speech get some manic patients into trouble. Many also get into trouble because their poor judgment and grandiosity or inflated self-esteem lead to significant social or economic problems. Manics tend to go on spending sprees, undertake foolish business ventures, drive recklessly, or travel on impulse to faraway places. For example, one manic patient, who had been a successful real-estate dealer and insurance salesman, decided to expand his business to Hawaii. He purchased a plane, hired four pilots to fly it, took all his employees with him to set up an office in Honolulu, wrote a series of bad checks, and ended up deeply in debt. Although he had no insight at the time of his illness, when asked afterward if he really needed four pilots, he replied ruefully, "Heavens, no. I didn't need any pilots. I didn't need an office in Honolulu. I didn't even need an airplane ticket."

In some patients, manic grandiosity may approach delusional proportions. A manic patient may believe he has special communication with God, a unique mission in life, or unusual powers, knowledge, or abilities. For example, one manic patient of modest means and a rural background was hospitalized by his disconcerted wife after he declared himself divorced from her by divine dispensation, flew to Miami, and waited there for several days for Jackie Kennedy to join him. He believed it was God's will that he would be declared King of Nations and Jackie Queen of Nations. Together they would rule the world from their headquarters in Miami Beach.

Some manics have rapid shifts in mood from elation to anger or depression. The anger may make them quite difficult to deal with. Manics hate to be contradicted or to have their various grandiose plans thwarted. Because they feel so good and have very little insight about the risks of their illness, they may resist treatment or hospitalization even when it is badly needed. Yet such patients may require protection from the consequences of their poor judgment or overactivity. In fact, before modern treatments for mania were available, it was a life-threatening illness: Approximately 15 percent of manic patients died from physical exhaustion. Even in the era of modern treatment, the excessive activity level continues to be a serious risk in patients with cardiac problems.

Yet another risk in mania is the possibility of a rapid switch to depression. Because many manics are truly "bipolar," they are particularly susceptible to the development of depression. Some may shift rapidly between mania and depression. Psychiatrists call these people "rapid cyclers." Others experience depression weeks or months after recovering from mania, while a few never develop significant symptoms of depression. When the manic patient becomes depressed, he is at a high risk for suicide, just as any other depressed person is, and the risk may be heightened in bipolar patients because the manic who has become depressed develops a remorseful insight into the folly of his previous manic behavior.

On the positive side, most manics tend to recover fully and to remain well between episodes. Maintenance lithium therapy is often prescribed (and will be discussed in more detail in chapter 8); it frequently prevents subsequent relapses or diminishes their severity. Further, many manic patients tend to be interesting, energetic, hardworking, and successful people. Bipolar illness may have a particularly close association with creativity and inventiveness. Martin Luther, Vincent van Gogh, and Robert Lowell are examples of particularly successful or creative people who have had bipolar illness. Some of these people, when treated with modern therapies, have expressed the insight that manic illness is crippling rather than liberating and that treatment has enhanced their capacity to be creative.

The Schizophrenic Disorders

When people think of "mental illness" or "being crazy," they are usually thinking of some form of schizophrenia. The person who walks along the street looking rather disheveled and muttering to himself is typically a schizophrenic. So is the person who is suspicious, defensive, and thinks people are after him and trying to harm or persecute him. Some schizophrenics, in spite of their illness, have enough charisma to convince other people of their delusional beliefs. Jim Jones, the leader of the Jonestown Massacre, was probably a schizophrenic. Some schizophrenics live in a fantasy world, absorbed in unreal relationships with people they scarcely know, but unable to have real relationships with people who are actually close to them, such as members of their own family. Such was the case with John Hinckley. Very infrequently schizophrenics may commit violent crimes, as did Hinckley and David Berkowitz. Since these violent crimes tend to get a great deal of attention from the media, people sometimes get the erroneous idea that most schizophrenics are violent. Usually they are not, although they tend to be quite unpredictable.

Schizophrenia is often a very crippling disease. Thus, while one can name many famous people who have suffered from affective disorders, it is much more difficult to name famous people who clearly suffered from schizophrenia. Nijinsky is a vivid example, but there are few others. Most people who develop schizophrenia do so at a relatively young age, and their intellectual and emotional capacities deteriorate steadily and inexorably as the disease progresses. That is why Kraepelin, when he first identified and defined the disease, called it "dementia praecox"—a dementing illness occurring in young people. Although we now know that not all schizophrenics deteriorate into dementia, particularly with the modern somatic therapies that are available, most people suffering from schizophrenia have some mental and emotional handicap and are unable to function at a high level.

Although schizophrenia is not as common as the affective disorders, it is nevertheless very common. Approximately 1 person in 100 suffers from schizophrenia. If that number seems small in comparison with the 8–20-percent rate for affective disorders, bear in mind that schizophrenia is usually a chronic illness rather than an episodic one. People with affective disorder become depressed or manic, are treated, recover, and go on about the business of their lives. They may never have another episode, or they may have several, but they are usually not chronically incapacitated.

The schizophrenic, on the other hand, tends to remain chronically ill. He may have periods of feeling worse or feeling better, but even at his best he is usually not the same person he was before he became ill. In the language of psychiatry, "schizophrenics rarely return to their premorbid level of functioning." That is why schizophrenia is a far more serious illness than affective disorder. People who have it tend to pile up in mental hospitals. It has been estimated that 30 percent of the hospital beds (*all* hospital beds—not just psychiatric beds) in the United States are occupied by people suffering from schizophrenia. Patients who are not hospitalized are often unable to work. Consequently, they frequently receive Social Security disability benefits. The economic, personal, and social costs of schizophrenia are high indeed.

Further, although it is difficult to identify many famous people who have schizophrenia, it does not spare the families of the great. James Joyce's daughter had schizophrenia. So did Bertrand Russell's daughter. Whether famous or not, watching one's child suffer the varied and painful symptoms of schizophrenia is an anguishing experience for parents, who often go from one doctor to another, hoping for a miracle cure. None exists at the moment. The psychiatrist who either discovers a definitive treatment for schizophrenia or identifies the major factors causing it will perhaps make the most important medical contribution of the twentieth century. When that happens, the impact on the lives of its victims and their relatives will be as great as when insulin was synthesized and used as a treatment for diabetes. Solving the riddle of schizophrenia is the single most important research goal in psychiatry today. Many clues are already available, enough to indicate that the solution will probably be discovered within our lifetime, perhaps even within the next ten to twenty years.

The most common misconception about schizophrenia is that it means "split personality." The syndrome of multiple personalities, which was portrayed in *The Three Faces of Eve,* is extremely rare and quite different from true schizophrenia. The term *schizophrenia* was coined by the Swiss psychiatrist Eugen Bleuler, who recognized that not all patients who had dementia praecox actually deteriorated into a demented state. He chose a new name, schizo-phrenia, to refer to the "splitting of the mind" that occurs in these patients. Although not all are demented, Bleuler believed that all had some disturbance in their ability to think clearly, to feel normally, and to act decisively.

Schizophrenia is a very complicated illness, and patients suffering from it may be very different from one another. Some may be bothered primarily by hallucinations, others by disturbances in their thinking, and others by an abnormality of emotional responsiveness. Further, the symptoms in any individual patient may change over the course of time. The following are two case histories of very different forms of schizophrenia.

Eileen Abbott is at present a thirty-eight-year-old married woman. If one were to meet her, one would not notice anything obviously wrong with her. Nevertheless, she has had a diagnosis of schizophrenia and has been handicapped by this illness since her early twenties.

Her early childhood and teen-age years were unremarkable, although she was considered somewhat shy and moody. The first hint of a problem occurred when she left home to attend college at a midwestern state university. She was living in a dormitory, as was required of all first-year students, and planning to obtain a degree in nursing. She began to call home to her parents quite frequently, expressing a concern that the dormitory was "not safe." Her parents became concerned and asked for more details but were given only vague replies such as "It's just a funny feeling I have," or "I'm just not sure I can trust everyone here." Her parents attributed her complaints to "separation anxiety" and the stress of attending college. When she returned home for Christmas vacation, however, they observed that she had lost some of her spontaneity and had undergone a noticeable personality change. She seemed preoccupied, worried, and even a bit aloof. She was guarded in her descriptions of college life. As far as they could tell, she did not seem to have found any close friends. She was able to finish her first year at the state university, but her grades were much lower than her past academic performance would have predicted, since she had been a nearly straight A student in high school and had obtained high scores on her SATs.

After the end of her first year, her parents suggested that she transfer to a small private college closer to her home, hoping this would ease some of the worry and unhappiness that she so obviously displayed. Instead, however, the problems became markedly worse during her second year in college. Now she lived only fifty miles from her parents, and she would drive home each weekend to see them. She began to talk with them somewhat more openly, expressing fears that the other students were "out to get" her. As she described some of the evidence supporting this feeling, her parents were astonished at her suspiciousness and tendency to overinterpret minor events. For example, she was unable to find her car keys one day, and she was convinced that her dormitory counselor had taken them and hidden them in order to prove to her that she "needed to be more free." One day when an instructor announced an upcoming midterm exam, he smiled and said they should expect it to be difficult and should not plan to rely on reviewing lecture notes alone. She interpreted this as a special warning that was being given to her and to her only, and took it as an indication that the administration expected her to flunk out. When she walked into a classroom or the dining room, she frequently felt that people had just been talking about her and laughing at her. She stayed up very late, studied constantly, and avoided social contact with her fellow students. Her parents continued to try to believe that she was having trouble handling the stress of college.

Finally, one day an incident occurred that was impossible to explain away on this basis. Eileen had come home for a weekend in late spring. She seemed particularly anxious and worried when she arrived. By late Sunday afternoon, when she was due to return, she was tearful, tremulous, and pacing up and down. Eventually she confessed that she was certain that someone was going to take her life if she returned. She had been hearing a warning voice, which was an unfamiliar male voice, telling her, "Don't go back. Don't go back." She felt that several of the students were playing "mind games" with her and were controlling her thoughts and actions. For example, even from the distance of fifty miles, she could feel them sending her messages and trying to draw her back like a magnet. She was convinced that when she arrived, she would be physically harmed in some way. Her parents called the dormitory counselor, who indicated that Eileen's fears were obviously unfounded and that Eileen had been behaving in a peculiar and suspicious manner for a number of months, arousing concern in some of the residents that she was having some type of psychiatric problem. Several people, including the counselor, had urged her to see a doctor at Student Health, but she was unwilling to do so. Her parents took her to a local psychiatrist, who recommended hospitalization.

Eileen was treated with neuroleptic medication (also called "antipsychotics") and was in the hospital for only three weeks. After discharge, she seemed to be nearly back to her old self. She returned to college and finished the semester.

During the next several years, Eileen was able to finish college, obtain a degree in nursing, and become married. The doctor who cared for her tried to discontinue her medication after about six months, but each time he tried, she began to show symptoms of suspiciousness and fearfulness. Consequently, she continued to take the medication.

Problems arose again, however, when she became pregnant with her first child. Prior to the delivery, she became increasingly fearful again, and afterward she was confused, restless, and markedly delusional. She was convinced that people were trying to harm the baby in many different ways: His milk might be poisoned; the diapers might contain dangerous chemicals; evil spirits were making him cry; the next-door neighbor was practicing voodoo. In spite of her concern about the baby's welfare, she was completely inadequate in her care of him. For example, she was often unable to perform a task as simple as changing a diaper. She would begin to do it and then leave him on the counter and go out in the kitchen to check the milk in order to be sure that it was still "safe," not taking adequate precautions to ensure that he would not fall off. Increasingly concerned about both her welfare and the baby's, her husband insisted that she enter the hospital again three weeks after delivery.

While in the hospital, Eileen was placed on a higher dose of neuroleptic medication. After about four weeks, she began to show some improvement. She was eventually able to return home and to care for her child in a reasonably efficient manner. Over the next ten years, however, she had several additional episodes of becoming severely delusional and agitated and again required rehospitalization. In between these episodes, she was withdrawn and suspicious. She was unwilling to go out to parties, to entertain people in her home, or to go on family vacations. Her husband did his best to maintain the appearance of normal family life. He insisted that his wife keep her fears and suspicions to herself and not communicate them either to their children or to the neighbors. Nevertheless, she did so occasionally, making veiled references to the fact that their home was "under surveillance." She rarely smiled or even showed much spontaneity in talking with her children. Nevertheless, she dressed attractively, kept the house well organized and clean, prepared appropriate meals, and took some pleasure in her children's accomplishments as they grew up. Her husband's friends and neighbors considered her rather aloof and eccentric, and they knew she had "nervous breakdowns" from time to time. She has been taking medication continuously for the past twenty years. Any efforts to discontinue it always lead to a significant worsening of her symptoms.

Eileen has a somewhat less severe form of schizophrenia. Her principal symptom is delusional thinking. Initially this occurred only briefly and responded well to medication. Over the years, however, her delusions have become more entrenched and do not respond as well to medication. She has coped moderately well by learning not to discuss her strange ideas with anyone else. While her ability to relate emotionally to others has deteriorated as her illness has progressed, she has been able to function reasonably well as a mother and home-maker with considerable support and assistance from her husband.

Roger Wallis, on the other hand, illustrates a more severe type of schizophrenic illness.

> Roger Wallis is at present forty-two. He lives in a state hospital and has been there more or less continuously since the death of his last surviving parent five years ago.
>
> It is difficult to say when his problems really began. Even when he was a young child, his family noticed that he was extremely shy and rather withdrawn. Although he was clearly attached to them and depended on them when he was a young child, he did not enjoy hugging, kissing, and other expressions of affection the way the rest of their children did. When he entered school, he tended to be solitary. He was an average student, but his parents considered him bright and creative because he read a great deal, had a large vocabulary, and enjoyed various intellectual games such as crossword puzzles or math puzzles. He was also preoccupied with inventing things. While in high school, he invented a new alphabet that was supposed to be more phonetically functional than the one currently in use. Although he tried to explain its basic principles to a number of people, no one seemed able to understand it. For a time, his parents were unable to decide whether he was sometimes difficult to understand because he was so much smarter than they, or whether his thinking was simply disorganized.
>
> He completed high school with average grades. He did not participate in any school activities, had no friends, and never went out on a date. He began college, but dropped out with failing grades after the end of the first semester. He returned home and lived with his parents. In spite of repeated efforts to get him out of the house and into various types of jobs, ranging from library clerk to janitor, he was never able to persist and perform any task in a dependable manner. He became increasingly absorbed in a fantasy world and spent much of his time involved in "intergalactic communication." He received messages from an unknown galaxy in a special language that only he was able to understand. These messages, which he heard as if they

were voices talking to him inside his head, would describe events in the distant galaxy of Atan. While he was in his twenties, he appeared to enjoy telling his parents about Atan, its local politics, and the people who lived there.

As he grew older, however, he seemed to lose interest in discussing his inner world and his inner voices with anyone. Never very interested in his appearance, he became downright disheveled. He had to be encouraged by his parents to wear clean clothing, to bathe, and to shave. If left to his own devices, he tended to select rather bizarre attire and hairstyles. His preferred dress consisted of long underwear, overalls, and a baseball cap that he wore backwards and left on his head even when he was indoors.

His parents sought psychiatric care for Roger intermittently, beginning in childhood. He was evaluated by a child psychiatrist at age eight. The psychiatrist commented on the discrepancy between his large vocabulary and his extreme social immaturity. Testing at the time also indicated a marked unevenness of performance in various tests of mental and social functioning. The psychiatrist expressed concern about an early psychiatric problem but also held out the hope that he might outgrow some of these problems with the passage of time.

Roger was briefly hospitalized after he returned home from college. He was placed on medication, which seemed to help only minimally. His inability to follow through on tasks, extreme withdrawal, and preoccupation with his fantasy world seemed to proceed inexorably. After the death of his mother, when he was thirty-two, he again required hospitalization. Intensive doses of medication seemed to help temporarily, but then the withdrawal returned. His father died when he was thirty-six, and he tried to live at home alone for the next year. He was eventually rehospitalized after complaints from neighbors brought him to the attention of community agencies. He had been living in the house for the past year without ever having done the laundry, taken out the garbage, or washed the dishes. When he decided that his overalls were dirty, he simply threw them in a corner and bought another pair. The house was filled with rotting food, debris, and old newspapers. He has subsequently remained in the hospital, since he is not likely to be able to function when living alone.

Roger had many characteristics that suggest to psychiatrists that schizophrenia will have a severe and deteriorating course. First of all, he had a "poor premorbid adjustment." Even as a relatively small child, he did not show a normal capacity to feel and express affection for others. As he grew older, he did not have normal relationships with children his own age. Signs of illness began early in life, and they developed so slowly and insidiously that it is difficult to point to a particular time and say that he "became schizophrenic" at that time.

Second, after his illness was obvious, many of his prominent symptoms were what are called "negative" or "defect" symptoms, in contrast to "positive" or "florid" symptoms. Florid symptoms include delusions, hallucinations, and fluent but disorganized speech. Roger had some of these symptoms early in his illness, but his most prominent symptoms were "defect" ones such as his inability to follow through on tasks (avolition), inability to enjoy relationships with other people (asociality), and inability to feel and express emotions (affective blunting). While positive or florid symptoms tend to respond relatively well to medication, negative symptoms are more resistant to treatment. Consequently, doctors were able to do very little to help Roger. Had he not had parents who were willing to care for him for many years, he probably would have been chronically hospitalized much earlier—or, in the less socially benevolent parts of our country, he would have become a starving, confused, and victimized skid-row bum.

Each of these examples of schizophrenia is an oversimplification, in that neither describes fully the wide range of symptoms and outcomes that may occur in schizophrenia. Some schizophrenics do better than Eileen. Some have scattered episodes of illness and are almost symptom-free between them. This course, however, is relatively rare. Some schizophrenics are able to function at nonstressful jobs, particularly those that do not demand a great deal of contact with other people, such as library work or custodial work. Some are unemployed but are able to live in the community despite their handicap, through various social assistance programs. Some live in sheltered workshops or halfway houses.

As the above case histories indicate, many different kinds of symptoms occur in schizophrenia, making it more difficult to understand than are the affective disorders. The affective disorders are characterized by an underlying disturbance in mood, be it elation or depression. Schizophrenia is characterized by multiple symptoms that occur in different patterns in different patients.

Delusions and hallucinations are the most colorful kinds of symptoms. A delusion is defined as a "fixed false belief." Delusions of persecution (or paranoia) are perhaps the commonest kind. Eileen's persecutory delusions are fairly typical. A person suffering from persecutory delusions is often difficult to deal with because she is suspicious, guarded, and irritable or angry. One must remember that the person suffering from such delusions is living in a terrifying and painful world. Danger lurks around every corner, and almost anyone might be involved in the conspiracy. Because they frequently have intact, or nearly intact, emotional responsiveness, people with paranoid delusions often appear superficially to function relatively well, especially if they avoid discussing their delusions with others or if their delusions seem believable. Indeed, one sometimes suspects that occasionally paranoid individuals may even rise to positions of considerable power in the government, military, or religious establishments. Jim Jones was probably such a charismatic paranoid.

Delusions may also take other forms. Sometimes patients have grandiose delusions, such as believing that they have special abilities or powers, although this tends to occur more commonly in mania. Delusions may be religious in nature. Sometimes it is difficult to differentiate between a religious delusion and a religious belief. Friends, relatives, and doctors must always use the patient's religious and cultural background as an aid in deciding whether a particular religious idea is a pathological delusion or an understandable belief, as well as whether the religious idea improves the patient's ability to function or interferes with it. Sometimes delusions are fantastic or bizarre. Delusions of this type suggest a more severe or serious case of illness. Roger's delusions were clearly fantastic. Further types of bizarre delusions that occur fairly commonly in schizophrenia include the belief that thoughts are being planted in one's mind, the belief that thoughts are stolen from one's mind, the feeling that others can hear one's thoughts aloud, or the belief that one's feelings and actions are controlled by some alien or outside force.

People suffering from schizophrenia also frequently experience various kinds of hallucinations. Hallucinations are defined as abnormal perceptions, such as hearing voices, seeing visions, or experiencing unusual sensations in one's body. Hearing voices (auditory hallucination) is easily the most common kind. The voices may be familiar or unfamiliar, male or female, single or multiple. They may comment on what the patient is doing or make mocking and derisive remarks. Early in the illness, patients tend to find their voices troubling or annoying. After a few years, they may be less bothered by them. Various kinds of visual distortions sometimes occur early in schizophrenia. For example, sometimes patients experience their hands as being larger than usual or their penises as being smaller than usual. On the other hand, frank visual hallucinations, such as seeing visions of people who are not really there, are relatively uncommon in schizophrenia. When a person reports visual hallucinations, the cause is more likely to be some form of intoxication with drugs or alcohol than schizophrenia.

Patients with schizophrenia may tend to think or talk in a very disorganized manner. Sometimes this symptom is so severe that the patient makes no sense at all when he talks. For example, when asked what his favorite class in high school was, one patient replied:

> Let's see, there was one I would have liked if it wasn't for the instructor, well, I got along with him, he was always wanting me to do the worst in the class, it seemed like, and I'd always get bad, the grade, in my grading, and he tried to make other people like they were good enough to be in Hollywood or something, you know I'd be the last one down the ladder. That, that's the way they wanted the grading to be in the first place according to whose, theirs, they, they have all different reasons that I, I, I think that they use that they want one, won't come out. One of the social status of, ah, of how big and strong a baseball, football player could be, you know, and he'll, he'll come in beating down on his head with the bottom of his fist if he doesn't do it his way, you know. That's how the show goes. And another one is the pretty girls in there that try so hard, that try so hard to get their, their thoughts and their, their hierarchy, it was a recreational leadership thing, their leadership, their leadership got there before I could get mine in order that they, they could be the first with the, with the doctor, you know, I wasn't going to be real, really abrupt in trying to break in between them or trying to talk to the, the instructor because they, they would have started yelling at me, get out of the way, or something.

Sometimes patients talk at length and seem to be making sense for a time, but then lapse into vagueness and stock phrases. For example, in the process of describing himself, one patient said the following:

> If you judge from my speech that I think quite a bit, you're perfectly right. I do. I think a lot. And therefore I have benefit to myself by assuaging whatever doubts about myself I may have in the inclusion of a day perceived as the doubtless recognition of a question of comprehension of point of view or differentiation of a model of endeavor or comprehension of experience as considered a differentiation of a demonstration of an identity distinguished by a mode of understanding and development of a point of view. In other words, I'm the same person who likes to understand himself, understand his sexuality at the same time, without needing to interpret one into the other or another into the opposite range of interest distinguished by a model of understanding, the analysis of which is commensurated by a question or comprehension of existence. . . . In other words, I'm not psychotic. So that's another thing I don't do. I don't perform the psychotic ritual of escape from the world by demonstrating a sublimation of my sensibility from the recognition of experience.

Both these examples are tape-recorded transcriptions of actual speech made with the patients' knowledge and permission, and they are quite representative of their usual speech. The first was always incoherent, while the second made sense sometimes, and sometimes lapsed into vague stock phrases. Most schizophrenics do not sound this disorganized. In fact, patients who have the most severe disorganization in thinking tend to say little or nothing. Their replies are brief, vague, and usually uninformative. This is called "poverty of speech," or "alogia." The emptiness of their speech probably reflects an emptiness in their minds.

Delusions, hallucinations, and disorganized speech tend to occur early in the illness. As it progresses, these symptoms sometimes "burn out." The patient is then left only with prominent negative or defect symptoms. Looking at things superficially, one might think that a person is better off no longer hearing voices or feeling persecuted. Indeed, one might think the patient is better off once he has lost his capacity to feel intensely. But the "burned-out" schizophrenic is an empty shell—he cannot think, feel, or act. The schizophrenic who hears voices can hope that medication will drive away the voices and that he can return to a relatively normal life. The schizophrenic with defect symptoms has lost the capacity both to suffer and to hope—and at present, medicine has no good remedy to offer for this loss.

Anxiety Disorders

W. H. Auden has called ours the "Age of Anxiety." Like affective disorders, anxiety disorders are relatively common. It has been estimated that 2–8 percent of the population has at some time suffered from some type of anxiety disorder.

Unlike depression, a syndrome that has been recognized for centuries, the syndrome of anxiety has been recognized only in relatively recent times. A physician named DaCosta is usually given the credit for first describing anxiety disorders. He called them "irritable heart" in the *American Journal of Medical Sciences* in 1871. The patient he described was a soldier who developed the syndrome during the Civil War. Since chest pain, pounding heart, and dizziness were the main symptoms that the soldier complained of, DaCosta thought that the disorder was due to a psychologically induced cardiac disturbance characterized by excessive sensitivity in the nerves that control heart activity. One might say that Stephen Crane recognized the same syndrome in *The Red Badge of Courage,* providing us with a literary account of this illness. After DaCosta's report, doctors began to diagnose this syndrome in patients who were experiencing serious stress, such as during warfare. It has been called by various names, such as "soldier's heart," the "effort syndrome," or "neurocirculatory asthenia."

While internists and family doctors were emphasizing cardiovascular aspects of the anxiety syndrome, psychiatrists and neurologists were becoming more interested in its psychological aspects during the late nineteenth and early twentieth centuries. Freud was responsible for recognizing anxiety as the core symptom in the syndrome and for introducing the term *anxiety neurosis.* Freud's conceptualization brought the patient's inner subjective feelings to the forefront, emphasizing the sense of fearfulness, terror, panic, and impending doom.

Anxiety disorders are characterized by a mixture of physical and psychological symptoms, and doctors still do not agree about the relative importance of the symptoms and especially about which reflect the underlying cause. Typical physical symptoms of anxiety include a pounding heart, a rapid pulse, chest pain or tightness, difficulty catching one's breath even at rest, feelings of asphyxiation, sweating, blushing, tingling sensations in the hands, nausea, diarrhea, abdominal pain, tremulousness, dizziness, weakness, and a tendency to tire easily. The psychological symptoms include tension, nervousness, apprehensiveness, a tendency to startle easily, hyperalertness and excessive vigilance, and subjective feelings of terror or panic.

The relative relationship of these physical and psychological symptoms is still a matter of some debate. Early in this century, the noted philosopher and psychologist William James proposed that the psychological experience of anxiety is nothing more than an awareness of the physical symptoms of anxiety, thus implying that the physical experience is primary. Freud, on the other hand, believed that psychological anxiety was primary and led to the development of physical symptoms. Whichever is primary, once the symptoms have begun, the relationship is almost certainly interactive, with psychological anxiety sometimes triggering physical symptoms, and physical symptoms sometimes leading to psychological anxiety.

Nervousness and fear are common human emotions that nearly everyone has experienced at one time or another. Consequently, as in the case of differentiating depressive disorder from unhappiness, it is also important to distinguish between anxiety disorders and anxiety as a normal or adaptive response. Feeling anxious and fearful when being attacked by a grizzly bear is a normal response. Dangerous or life-threatening situations trigger reactions in the parts of the nervous system that govern the level of arousal and regulate blood flow to the parts of the body that need it most. These regulatory centers, called the "autonomic nervous system," prepare the person for what physicians call the "fight or flight" response. To a lesser degree, many people experience the same kind of anxiety, triggered by autonomic arousal, before taking an examination or giving a talk. In these cases, the anxiousness and hyperalertness are also normal and adaptive as long as the tension does not become excessive or handicapping. Even classic phobias, such as fear of heights or open spaces, may reflect some primitive adaptive response. Thus anxiety may be potentially quite useful to human beings in helping them cope with the stresses and threats of life. Anxiety should only be considered pathological, and therefore a symptom of a psychiatric disorder, when it ceases to be helpful or adaptive and instead becomes crippling or disabling.

The anxiety disorders are usually divided into three main groups. These are summarized in table 2. As the table indicates, the older term for these disorders is *neuroses,* the term that Freud used to describe them.

Table 2.
CLASSIFICATION OF ANXIETY DISORDERS

Phobic Disorders *(or Phobic Neuroses)*	*Anxiety States* *(or Anxiety Neuroses)*	*Post–Traumatic Stress* *Disorder*
Agoraphobia	Panic Disorder	Acute Post-Traumatic Stress Disorder
Social Phobia	Generalized Anxiety Disorder	Chronic Post-Traumatic Stress
Simple Phobia	Obsessive-Compulsive Disorder	Disorder

THE NATURE OF PHOBIC DISORDERS

The following case history illustrates a fairly typical example of one type of phobic disorder, agoraphobia (literally, fear of the market-place; more loosely, fear of going out).

> Greg Miller is a twenty-seven-year-old unmarried computer pro-grammer. When asked about his main problem, he replied, "I am afraid to leave my house or drive my car."
>
> The patient's problems began approximately one year ago. At that time he was driving across the bridge that he must traverse every day in order to go to work. While driving in the midst of the whizzing six-lane traffic, he began to think (as he often did) about how awful it would be to have an accident on that bridge. His small, vulnerable VW convertible could be crumpled like an aluminum beer can, and he could die a bloody, painful death or, still worse, be crippled for life. His car could even hurtle over the side of the bridge and plunge into the river.
>
> As he thought about these possibilities, he began to feel increas-ingly tense and anxious. He glanced back and forth at the cars on either side of him and became frightened that he might run into one of them. Then he experienced an overwhelming rush of fear and panic. His heart started pounding and he felt as if he were going to suffocate. He began to take deeper and deeper breaths, but this only increased his sense of suffocation. His chest felt tight and he won-dered if he might be about to die of a heart attack. He certainly felt that something dreadful was going to happen to him quite soon. He stopped his car in the far right lane in order to try to regain control of his body and his feelings. Traffic piled up behind him with many

honking horns, and drivers pulled around him yelling obscenities. On top of his terror, he experienced mortification. After about three minutes, the feeling of panic slowly subsided, and he was able to proceed across the bridge and go to work. During the remainder of the day, however, he worried constantly about whether or not he would be able to make the return trip home across the bridge without a recurrence of the same crippling fear.

He managed to do so that day, but during the next several weeks he would begin to experience anxiety as he approached the bridge, and on three or four occasions he had a recurrence of the crippling attack of panic. The panic attacks began to occur more frequently so that he had them daily. By this time he was overwhelmed with fear and began to stay home from work, calling in sick each day. He knew that his main symptom was an irrational fear of driving across the bridge, but he suspected that he might also have some type of heart problem. He saw his family doctor, who found no evidence of any serious medical illness, and who told him that his main problem was excessive anxiety. The physician prescribed a tranquilizer for him and told him to try to return to work.

For the next six months, Greg struggled with his fear of driving across the bridge. He was usually unsuccessful and continued to miss a great deal of work. Finally, he was put on disability for a few months and told by the company doctor to seek psychiatric treatment. Greg was reluctant and embarrassed to do this, and instead he stayed home most of the time, reading books, listening to records, playing chess on his Apple computer, and doing various "handyman" chores around the house. As long as he stayed home, he had few problems with anxiety or the dreadful attacks of panic. But when he tried to drive his car, even to the nearby shopping center, he would sometimes have panic attacks. Consequently, he found himself staying home nearly all the time and soon became essentially housebound. Finally, his parents (with whom he lived) became so concerned that they insisted he seek psychiatric treatment.

The patient is the youngest of four children. His father is a middle-level-management executive at the same company where Greg worked as a computer programmer. Greg and his two older sisters were always noted to be rather shy, sensitive children, while his older brother was gregarious and popular. All were good students. Greg had only one or two close friends as a child, and these tended to be boys who shared his bookish interests and his fascination with computers. He did not date in high school or college, and he always suspected that girls would not want to go out with him. Although he was neither strikingly handsome nor strikingly unattractive, he himself believed that he was scrawny and homely, and during his college years he grew a beard to cover up a chin that he considered "too weak." Nevertheless, Greg did not consider himself unhappy.

His life changed strikingly during his sophomore year in college. He and his older brother, Bill, both attended a small private school in Vermont. Bill was bright, outgoing, and had many friends. Greg admired and respected him. He recalls feeling no envy of his older brother's success, although he did occasionally wish that he could give his parents as much pleasure as Bill did.

On the last day of the second semester of his sophomore year, Greg returned to his dormitory room and found a small group of white-faced friends and acquaintances. They told him that Bill had been hit by a car while riding back from an exam on his bike. It had been a rainy day and Bill had been riding fast with his head down, not looking as carefully as he should. When bicycle and car collided, Bill was thrown twenty feet and died instantly. Greg had become his parents' only son. He found the responsibility to be heavy indeed.

Greg had difficulty returning to college the next fall. In fact, after the first few weeks, he found the surroundings too painful and decided to transfer to another school. This time he selected a large state university. He was a loner there but did well academically, graduating with honors. He then went on to obtain a master's degree in computer science, applied for a programming job at his father's firm, and was accepted. Rather than getting an apartment of his own, he decided to live with his parents for a while, rationalizing that it would permit him to save more money. His parents were away much of the time, but when home were friendly and supportive. They did urge him to go out a bit more—to join a church group, to meet more people his own age, and to try to find a girlfriend. As he became increasingly incapacitated by his anxiety and panic, they at first saw the problem as a possible natural consequence of his shyness and perhaps as a delayed psychological reaction to his brother's death. They thought it would eventually "work itself out" if they gave him plenty of encouragement and support. Finally, it became clear that the problem was not going to clear up spontaneously and that their son had a relatively serious mental illness.

Any psychiatrist would diagnose Greg's problem as agoraphobia, complicated by panic attacks. As is often the case with panic attacks, once they began, they led to a vicious cycle of retreat, followed by increasing fear, followed by even greater retreat. Like many people who experience intense anxiety, Greg became increasingly crippled until he was housebound. The treatment of such patients is difficult, since they are fearful of leaving the house even to obtain treatment! Some patients with panic attacks and agoraphobia respond remarkably well to medication and need little else in the way of treatment. Greg, however, was not one of those lucky people. His treatment persisted for several years and ranged from psychoanalytic psychotherapy to a variety of different medications. He appeared to respond best to a combined treatment that involved taking medications, learning to control his attacks of fear through systematic desensitization and relaxation training, and attending a support group whose membership consisted of other people suffering from agoraphobia.

Agoraphobia is probably the most common and most crippling of the various phobic disorders. All the phobias are characterized by a persistent and irrational fear of some stimulus, which leads to a compelling desire to avoid it. The agoraphobic has a fear of being alone or in public places from which he may be unable to escape. Typical situations that the agoraphobic fears include being in a crowd, driving on a busy street, or being in enclosed spaces such as tunnels, bridges, or elevators. Patients suffering from agoraphobia tend increasingly to restrict their activities in order to avoid the feared situation, and they often insist that a family member or friend accompany them whenever they leave home. In severe cases, patients may become housebound. Frequently, agoraphobia is accompanied by panic attacks. Sometimes psychological triggers can be found that may initially induce the panic attack. Greg's illness developed in an individual who had been psychologically primed both by his basically shy personality and by the unexpected violent death of his brother. Quite often, however, the clinician searches for such psychological triggers in vain. Once such psychological triggers can be found, some patients are assisted by psychotherapy that helps them understand and work through the underlying conflict. But others do not appear to be helped by such therapy.

Social and simple phobias involve more-circumscribed stimuli. Social phobia is a fear of situations in which the person is exposed to scrutiny or observation by others. Common social phobias include fear of public speaking, fear of eating in public, or fear of using public lavatories. Simple phobias include all other phobias, such as fear of animals or fear of heights. Usually the person fears that he or she will behave in a manner that may be humiliating or embarrassing, and this fear leads to "phobic avoidance." The person recognizes that these fears are excessive or unreasonable. Often the person's anticipatory anxiety leads to impaired performance in the feared situation, as when a person with a fear of public speaking forgets what she wanted to say or speaks in a tremulous voice. When beginning the speech, the person may experience symptoms of panic, such as tachycardia or shortness of breath. Thus, psychological factors (anticipatory anxiety) interact with physical factors (tremulousness, tachycardia) and environmental stresses (giving a speech) to set up a vicious interactive cycle that perpetuates the disorder.

THE NATURE OF ANXIETY STATES

Phobic disorders all involve fear of some specific stimulus, whether it be a situation such as being in a crowd, or a specific object such as dogs or snakes. They are equivalent to the older concept of phobic neurosis. The anxiety states share the common thread of irrational anxiety, but the anxiety is not tied to a specific stimulus. They correspond to the older concept of anxiety neurosis. Modern systems of classification divide these anxiety states into three main groups: panic disorder, generalized anxiety disorder, and obsessive-compulsive disorder.

Panic disorder is characterized by recurrent attacks of anxiety or panic. Greg started out with panic disorder, but his condition eventually became so severe that he was given the more severe diagnosis of agoraphobia with panic attacks. A panic attack involves the sudden onset of a characteristic set of symptoms, such as shortness of breath, pounding heart, chest pain or discomfort, choking or smothering sensations, dizziness, numbness and tingling in the hands, trembling, sweating, and a feeling of impending doom. These attacks usually last only a few minutes, but in rare cases they may last for hours. Many normal people have experienced occasional panic attacks. If one describes a typical panic attack to a room full of 100 people and then asks how many have ever experienced anything like that (as I do each year with a group of medical students), one usually sees fifteen or twenty hands stick up in the air. The experience of having panic attacks becomes panic disorder when the attacks occur frequently and when a person begins to suffer some kind of significant discomfort or disability because of them.

Generalized anxiety disorder is less specific and often less serious than panic disorder. In fact, the classification that psychiatrists have developed for the anxiety disorders is usually hierarchical—that is, the more specific (and severe) disorders take diagnostic precedence over the less specific (less severe) ones. Although patients with agoraphobia, for example, may experience panic attacks when alone or in public places, they are not given the double diagnosis of phobic disorder and panic disorder; instead, the diagnosis of agoraphobia with panic attacks takes precedence. Likewise, patients who have frequent panic attacks may also experience generalized anxiety between panic attacks, but if the panic attacks are frequent, then the diagnosis of panic disorder is given precedence.

Thus, generalized anxiety disorder is an illness characterized by pervasive and persistent anxiety, but without phobias, panic attacks, or obsessions and compulsions. The patient simply feels anxious much of the time. Typical symptoms include motor tension (e.g., restlessness, shakiness, inability to relax), hyperactivity of the autonomic nervous system (e.g., sweating, pounding heart, dry mouth), apprehensive expectation (e.g., worry, fear), and excessive vigilance (e.g., insomnia, hyperalertness with distractibility, irritability). Patients who have these symptoms tend to have them relatively chronically. Many report that they seem to have been "born that way."

Obsessive-compulsive disorder is classified among the anxiety disorders because of the anxiety symptoms that develop whenever an individual attempts to resist an obsession or compulsion. An obsession is a persistent troubling thought that the person recognizes as senseless but is unable to get rid of. Common obsessions include a mother's fear that she may grab a knife and stab her child, a preoccupation with urinating in public, or thoughts about some type of inappropriate sexual behavior. A compulsion is a senselessly repetitive act. Common compulsions include handwashing, counting, checking, and touching. People who suffer from obsessions and compulsions tend to be conscientious, hardworking, gentle, and perhaps a bit rigid. They never act on their obsessions and actually do the thing they are preoccupied with. Sometimes, however, obsessive-compulsive disorder can become very severe and cause a person to be completely handicapped. The following is an example of such a case.

Liz Antonelli is a thirty-two-year-old unmarried woman who lives alone in her own apartment and is unemployed. She receives financial assistance from Social Security disability and from her parents. She takes a few classes at the local college and is slowly working toward a master's degree in library science.

Liz was first noticed to have problems at age eight, when her parents left her and her two older brothers with a baby-sitter in order to take a three-week vacation in Europe. Liz, always a somewhat worried and overconscientious child, became intensely preoccupied with the possibility that her mother might die while away on the vacation trip. Liz felt that if her mother died, she would somehow be responsible for it. She quickly developed a set of rituals that she believed might prevent her mother's death. At first she tried reading the first chapter of the Book of Genesis in a softly audible voice to herself each morning and evening upon arising and before going to bed. If she made any mistake, she would have to go to the beginning and start over until she was sure she had done it "just right." Soon this task began to take an hour or two each morning and evening. When the baby-sitter tried to make her stop in the morning so that she could attend school, Liz would cry, resist, and insist that "something terrible will happen" if she were made to stop reading. The baby-sitter let her miss the first few hours of school on several occasions, but eventually decided that she must force Liz to go to school. Liz cried hysterically during the entire car ride and was sent home in the afternoon by the school nurse. At dinner, the baby-sitter noticed that Liz was beginning to take a long time to get through the meal. Liz explained that she had to chew each bite precisely ten times or else "something terrible might happen." The baby-sitter also noticed that Liz's hands had become red and cracked. Liz explained that she had to wash them frequently to prevent them from becoming dirty and having a bad effect on other people.

When Liz's parents returned home, Liz's fears did not seem to diminish, despite her mother's ebullient good health. Liz continued to worry that she might somehow cause her mother's death if she did not continue her rituals. Her parents took her to a child psychiatrist, who eventually managed to get Liz to explain why she felt obliged to go through so many complicated rituals. The psychiatrist saw Liz once a week for about a year and helped her discuss her fears through the use of play therapy. With this treatment, Liz's rituals diminished and she was able to attend school on a regular basis. Her family was relieved by the improvement, but continued to worry about Liz's rigidity and excessive concern with order. Liz had to sit on the same chair every day at breakfast and dinner, and she would sometimes become upset at school if she were moved to a different seat in the classroom. Although she no longer took hours to get up in the morning or to go to bed at night, she was still slow and seemed to have to complete many more steps than did her two older brothers. She kept her books, clothes, and shoes in a very precise order and became disturbed if her mother or the cleaning lady moved them.

Liz continued in this mode of stable instability throughout the remainder of grade school, junior high school, and most of high school. She was an exceptional student who obtained top grades in nearly every course that she took. Her parents sometimes felt concerned that she spent so much time researching and writing term papers or preparing for exams. She was rather shy and had only one or two close friends. She preferred to spend most of her time reading books rather than going to football games or school proms. Her parents would often urge her to get out and do more, but she resisted.

At the end of Liz's senior year in high school, her parents planned the first major vacation trip that they had taken since the ill-fated one some ten years earlier. This was to be a second trip to Europe to visit the places they had not seen previously. They asked Liz to come along, but she preferred to remain home in order to review foreign languages and get ready for admission to college in the fall. Because of her excellent academic standing and her high SAT scores, she had been admitted to a very selective eastern girls' school. Her parents debated as to whether they could leave her home alone, but finally concluded that they could. Liz expressed some apprehension during the week or two prior to their departure, but seemed to respond well to reassurances and to a list of each hotel where they would be staying along with its phone number. As it turned out, their trip to Europe was punctuated by almost nightly phone calls from Liz to check on their welfare. The phone bill was nearly the size of their airfare. They returned home to find Liz badly decompensated. Although she had been left with the family car and ample funds to buy food and gas, after the first few days she had not left the house and had become almost completely incapacitated by reading, writing, eating, dressing, and washing rituals.

Instead of entering college that fall, Liz entered a psychiatric hospital. The rituals did not improve after her parents' return and even after regular outpatient psychiatric therapy. Instead, she was almost totally helpless. The rituals seemed to get worse rather than better. She spent almost every minute of the day doing things and then undoing them. She could not button her clothes because she never had them "quite right," and she would have to take them off, put them on, and start buttoning all over again. Just getting dressed in the morning was a major task. She had similar reading rituals to those she had earlier. Now, however, she had to stop and count to ten every time she made a mistake, in addition to starting over again. She was preoccupied with the number ten, which tended to pervade all her rituals. Even poor Liz could not explain the reason for all this behavior, except for the fear that some harm would come to her family if she did not do it.

During the subsequent fourteen years, Liz had an up-and-down course. Her first psychiatric hospitalization lasted nearly a year. She received intensive psychotherapy in a private hospital, but was discharged with only minimal improvement. She then sought treatment at a university hospital facility, where she remained about six months. The treatment there consisted of behavior modification and medication. She responded somewhat better to this and was able to be discharged and to begin attending classes at the local state university. She took eight years to finish a four-year course load, but was able to graduate with a major in English. She had approximately five additional psychiatric hospitalizations during this time and clearly remained somewhat handicapped by her rituals and anxiety. In addition to feeling that she might bring harm to her family, she also began to suffer from an intense fear of failure in her university course work.

After she finally graduated from college at age twenty-six, her family insisted that she "pull herself together" and try to obtain a job. They felt that she had become too dependent on her psychiatrist at the university hospital, who had seen her continuously during that eight-year period. They insisted that she needed a "change of scenery" and requested that she go live with an aunt in Chicago, who would help her find a job. Liz did not respond at all well to this rather abrupt severance of her ties with her immediate family and her doctor. Her rituals, which had never completely disappeared, worsened markedly and she was again totally incapacitated. Eventually she was returned to the university hospital setting.

Although she continued to receive more or less the same treatment to which she had responded previously, this time Liz did not respond. She simply could not survive at all outside a protective hospital setting, in spite of repeated patient attempts to discharge her and to help her live independently. After two years of nearly continuous hospitalization, her doctors decided to treat her with cingulotomy, a form of psychosurgery that involves cutting a few fiber tracts in the cingulate gyrus of the brain (a technique described in more detail in chapter 8). Liz seemed to respond relatively well to this treatment. She was at least able to leave the hospital, live on her own, and return to school in order to try to obtain a master's degree. Most of her rituals disappeared gradually during the first six months after the surgery. However, she continued to be an overconscientious, over-self-disciplined, rigid, and relatively shy person. She is due to obtain her master's degree in library science within one year, and her doctors are hopeful that she will then be able to become self-employed.

Fortunately, such severe obsessive-compulsive disorder is quite rare. Unfortunately, it is also exceedingly difficult to treat. Some patients respond well to either psychotherapy or medications such as tricyclic antidepressants. When the illness has been completely disabling for many years, psychosurgery is sometimes used, as it was in Liz's case.

POST-TRAUMATIC STRESS DISORDER

Post-traumatic stress disorder is both a very old and a very new form of anxiety disorder. Since the first description of anxiety disorder, DaCosta's syndrome, was a case of anxiety occurring during the stress of combat, one might say that post-traumatic stress disorder has been recognized for a long time. On the other hand, it was not included in the official psychiatric classification system until quite recently.

Post-traumatic stress disorder is of current popular interest because a substantial number of cases appear to have been triggered by the stress of the Vietnam War. Ever since DaCosta, people have recognized that participating in warfare often leads to severe chronic anxiety both during combat and after the combat situation is over. Older terms include *shell shock, battle fatigue, traumatic war neurosis,* and *gross stress reaction.* This disorder also occurs after other catastrophic stressors, such as natural disasters, concentration camps, and large-scale accidents. Hiroshima, Dachau, and DC-10 crashes are all examples of psychologically traumatic events that are outside the range of usual human experiences and likely to lead to a post-traumatic stress disorder in some people.

People who experience these traumatic events typically relive them in a variety of ways, such as in recurrent dreams or nightmares, painful intrusive recollections, or suddenly acting or feeling as if the event were occurring again. They also suffer from something called "psychic numbing" or "emotional anesthesia." They complain of feeling detached, losing their capacity to enjoy themselves, or losing the ability to feel at all. They also develop symptoms of excessive autonomic arousal, such as hyperalertness, trouble falling asleep, or an exaggerated startle response. People who have shared life-threatening experiences with others, such as survivors of concentration camps, sometimes develop painful guilt feelings about surviving when others did not. They tend to avoid situations that make them recollect the trauma.

The novel *Sophie's Choice* provides a powerful literary portrayal of post-traumatic stress disorder in a death-camp victim. The following is an example of a typical case history of post-traumatic stress disorder occurring after combat.

> Jim Griggs is a twenty-six-year-old married Vietnam veteran recently laid off from a job he had held for three years. He was admitted to the hospital for severe symptoms of anxiety, which began after he was laid off at work and found himself at home watching reports of the fall of South Vietnam on TV. When asked what was wrong with him, he replied, "I don't know. I just can't seem to control my feelings. I'm scared all the time by my memories." Jim described himself as well adjusted and outgoing prior to his service in Vietnam. He was active in sports during high school. He was attending college part-time and working part-time to pay his way when he was drafted to serve in Vietnam. Although he found killing to be repulsive initially, he gradually learned to tolerate it and to rationalize it. He had several experiences that he found particularly painful and troubling. One of these occurred when he was ambushed by a Vietnamese

guerrilla, found his gun had jammed, and was forced to kill his enemy by bludgeoning him over the head repeatedly. Many years later he could still hear the "gook's" screams. Another extremely painful incident occurred when his closest friend was killed by mortar fire. Since they were lying side by side, the friend's blood splattered all over the patient.

Although he had some difficulty adjusting during the first year after his return from Vietnam, drifting aimlessly around the country in *Easy Rider* fashion and finding it difficult to focus his interests or energies, he eventually settled down, obtained a steady job, and married. He was making plans to return to college at the time he was laid off. At home with time on his hands, watching the fall of Vietnam on TV, he began to experience unwanted intrusive recollections of his own Vietnam experiences. In particular, he was troubled by the memory of the "gook" he had killed and the death of his friend. He found himself ruminating about all the people who were killed or injured and wondering what the purpose of it all had been. He began to experience nightmares, during which he relived the moments when he himself was almost injured. During one nightmare, he "dived for cover" out of bed and sustained a hairline fracture of the humerus. Another time he was riding his bike on a path through tall grass and weeds, which suddenly reminded him of the terrain in Vietnam, prompting him to dive off the bike for cover, and causing several lacerations to his arms and legs when he hit the ground. He also became increasingly irritable with his wife, and was admitted to the hospital because of her concern about his behavior.

He was treated with antianxiety drugs and psychotherapy, during which he was encouraged to ventilate and to recall and live through his past experiences. He responded well to this treatment and was discharged after three weeks. He continued to see a therapist weekly for another two months. Six months later he was essentially symptom-free and had returned to college.

Like many Vietnam veterans, Jim's predominant symptoms involved reliving, reexperiencing, and "flashback" episodes. During flashbacks, the reliving may be so intense that the patient acts as if he is actually reexperiencing the stressful event. Depending on the nature of the stressor, other symptoms may predominate in other patients. People who have lived through death camps or concentration camps may have more "survival guilt" and loss of the ability to form normal attachments, as did Sophie Zawistoska. People who have sustained serious physical injury in addition to their psychological injury, such as people injured in large-scale mass catastrophes, may have many autonomic symptoms and difficulty remembering or concentrating.

The course of post-traumatic stress disorder is variable. Most people who have experienced a significant stressor (defined as outside the range of normal human experience) tend to have an acute reaction. Quite frequently, however, this problem does not come to medical attention and clears spontaneously. In a few people, the reaction is more prolonged and becomes chronic. Sometimes, as in the case of Jim Griggs, the disorder erupts several years after the initial stressor. This is called a "delayed post-traumatic stress disorder." Post-traumatic stress disorder is not usually incapacitating, and it usually responds well to treatment. Most people who suffer from this disorder, even when it is relatively chronic, are able to work, but they may have some decrease in their ability to have normal interpersonal relationships. The outcome is usually worse when the initial stressor was especially prolonged and severe.

The Dementias

Schizophrenia—Kraepelin's dementia praecox—is a disease characterized by intellectual and emotional deterioration beginning at a relatively young age. The dementias have similar symptoms, but begin considerably later in life—usually sometime after age forty, typically in the fifties, sixties, or seventies. They are characterized by a loss of intellectual abilities, especially memory; emotional shallowness and lability; and personality change. In the beginning, these changes are often very subtle. The patient may notice that the symptoms are occurring and be quite distressed by them. Later, as the symptoms worsen, the patient may begin to lose insight about them. The following is a typical case history of a person suffering from dementia.

When first seen by a psychiatrist, Alice Fuhrmeister was a sixty-two-year-old housewife, mother of three, and grandmother of seven.

She was brought in for evaluation by her husband, who stated, "I just can't handle her anymore. For some reason, she has become a changed person." The patient herself said, "I don't know what's happened to me. I just can't remember anything anymore."

Prior to the onset of the present symptoms, Alice had had a relatively uneventful homelife. She grew up in a small New England town where her father prospered as the owner of the local grocery store. She was the eldest child and a family favorite. After completing high school, she left home for the university, met her present husband, and married him shortly after they both graduated. While the early years of their marriage were partially troubled by the Great Depression and World War II, they were nevertheless a happy couple. Although Alice was qualified to be a high-school science teacher, she chose not to work, devoting herself wholeheartedly to being a homemaker, as her mother had been. As her three children were born, Alice's life became increasingly involved with the home and family. Her husband noted with pride that when he came home from work each day the children were always dressed in neatly ironed clothes, with their hair nicely parted and their white shoes polished. As the children grew older, Alice spent many hours reading to them, helping them with their homework, driving them and their friends to school events, and keeping their rooms and clothes immaculately clean. She was a storybook mother who baked homemade cookies, delighted in clean laundry, and beamed with pride as her children blossomed into maturity.

Nevertheless, when their youngest child married and moved to another city shortly before Alice's fiftieth birthday, she began to seem slightly changed and somewhat depressed. All three children had grown into successful adults. Alice could claim two doctors and one lawyer among her offspring. Each child had chosen to move to another city to practice, and so Alice suddenly found herself with an "empty nest." Her husband worried as he observed her lose interest in church activities, sewing, and even homemaking. Both Alice and her husband tried to remedy the situation by spending more time with one another, taking long-postponed vacations together and sharing hobbies such as playing golf with friends and stamp collecting.

These measures helped somewhat, but Alice continued to change. Always remarkably even-tempered, she began to be more irritable. She would occasionally vent her feelings in angry outbursts at her husband, blaming him for the fact that the children had all moved away and no longer seemed to pay much attention to them. Her husband was steadily more perplexed, for he felt that someone who loved her children as much as Alice obviously did should be rejoicing in their success and happiness rather than resenting it. Always very much a lady, Alice began to swear occasionally, as she had never done previously. On one occasion at a luncheon after church, she went into a most uncharacteristic tirade among their close friends, complaining about the minister's sermon and calling him "nothing but a damned alcoholic." The minister tippled a bit, it was true, but Alice had tolerated this for the past ten years with equanimity. She also began to misplace things and frequently accused her husband of moving her things or even throwing them away.

When Alice was sixty, a major change occurred in her life and marriage. Her sixty-four-year-old husband, on whom she had been economically and socially dependent since the early years of her marriage, developed cancer of the larynx. His larynx was removed, leaving him with a markedly impaired ability to communicate. The doctors held out hope that all the cancer had been removed and that Harold would be able to live for many years. Alice was, nevertheless, surprisingly disconsolate. Harold retired from work and remained home with her. Alice became increasingly frustrated about having to live continuously with "an invalid." Although Harold did his best to try to hold things together, their storybook marriage deteriorated into disaster. Alice became increasingly preoccupied with various grievances that she felt she had experienced and spent hours berating her husband angrily about these. He was able to say a little in reply through "esophageal speech," but he was not able to say enough to reason with her. Making matters worse, Alice was becoming increasingly hard-of-hearing. Her evaluation by the psychiatrist was precipitated by a terrible quarrel one evening, which culminated when Alice grabbed a heavy fire poker from the fireplace and threatened to hit Harold over the head with it.

At the evaluation, Alice was noted to be a sweet-faced, gray-haired woman who looked somewhat older than her actual age. Harold, in spite of his surgery two years earlier, appeared exuberantly healthy. Nevertheless, he was clearly worried about his wife, wondering what was happening to her and to him. After an extensive evaluation of Alice's intellectual functions, it became clear that she had a significant impairment in memory and performed much worse on IQ testing than would a woman who had graduated from college. A CT scan suggested that her brain was somewhat atrophied, and an electro-encephalogram showed diffuse slow activity.

These findings led to a tentative diagnosis of Alzheimer's disease, a type of dementia that is steadily progressive and for which there is no known treatment. When this was explained to Harold, he resolved to take Alice home and take care of her as patiently as he could. He explained to the doctor: "I married her for better or worse. I've had the better, and now I guess I should try to take care of the worse."

The next several years became steadily more difficult, however. Alice's mind and personality seemed to recede farther and farther away. She was steadily more forgetful and could not be left alone in the kitchen because she would forget to turn off burners, to take food out of the oven, or to even turn off the running water. She overflowed the bathtub several times, forgetting that she had left it filling, and causing a major plaster and water avalanche from the second to the first story. Although her memory for recent events was poor, she did spend hours reminiscing about the past, reliving her childhood, the early years of her marriage, and her children's early years. She was frequently immature and childlike. In addition to many angry out-bursts toward Harold and toward her children and grandchildren when they phoned or visited, Alice also got into petty quarrels with the neighbors. Sometimes Harold would find her in the backyard shouting obscenities to neighborhood dogs or children. She got lost several times when she went outside for a walk. Once in the winter she wandered quite far from home attired only in a nightgown and bathrobe in subzero weather. She was unable to give her address or phone number to the policemen who finally found her, although she was able to remember her name.

Finally, very reluctantly, when Alice was sixty-seven, Harold concluded that he had to place her in a nursing home. She lived there until her death at age seventy. During the last year she did not even recognize members of her immediate family.

Like the other major psychiatric illnesses, the dementias are relatively common. Alzheimer's disease affects approximately 15 percent of people over age sixty-five. Other types of dementia, such as Huntington's chorea, are considerably rarer. Parkinson's disease, which affects approximately 2 percent of the population, is sometimes accompanied by dementia, although it is somewhat milder than the dementia of Alzheimer's disease.

Alice Fuhrmeister's history illustrates many of the features of dementia. During the early years of its development, its symptoms tend to be subtle and relatively mild. Often they are quite similar to those of depression, and early dementia is frequently misdiagnosed as depression. No harm is done when this occurs, except that family members are spared an early warning of impending misery. Patients with early mild dementia that is misdiagnosed as depression do not usually improve much with treatment, however, and the diagnosis eventually makes itself clear during subsequent years since the patient has the steady downhill deterioration so characteristic of the dementias.

The core symptom of dementia is impairment in mental functioning, especially memory loss. As in Alice's case, the oldest memories are usually spared during the early years of the illness, and most of the loss is in more recent memories. Patients misplace keys, lock themselves out of cars and houses, forget the names of people they have met, or fail to register checks. As the illness worsens, more-distant memories begin to go, and the names of old friends or even grandchildren are forgotten. Finally, like Alice, the patient is unable to recall her own address or phone number, and ultimately even her birth date or name.

The loss of intellectual function is usually accompanied by the loss of emotional functions. These symptoms were particularly prominent in Alice's case, as she underwent a personality change from being relatively placid and loving to being difficult, irritable, and labile. Sometimes patients become quite suspicious and distrustful. At other times they become shallow and inappropriate, laughing or making jokes in somber circumstances. These changes in emotion and personality are particularly difficult for friends and relatives, who feel that they are no longer dealing with the person they used to know and love.

Social judgment is also impaired. A man who was once quite proper may begin to make obscene overtures to young women or leave his fly unzipped without apparently caring. People who were formerly relatively modest about physical privacy will leave blinds up when they undress or wander outside in their pajamas or underwear. Interest in grooming and apparel disappears, and if unattended, patients will have unkempt hair, bathe infrequently, and forget to brush their teeth.

Just as the parents of a young person suffering from schizophrenia have the sense that a loved one is disappearing before their eyes, so, too, the spouses and children of patients with dementia look on these changes with grief, despair, and terror. Watching a loved one die of cancer is heartbreaking, but watching a loved one die slowly from dementia is even worse, for the loved one becomes almost totally unreachable. The person continues to live on, but with only vestiges and traces of her former self, and most of these are physical rather than mental or psychological. Dementia is a living death. Unless a cure or treatment is found, at least 10 percent of the readers of this book will experience it through developing the disease themselves.

5

THE REVOLUTION IN NEUROSCIENCE:

What Is the Brain?

> Men ought to know that from the brain, and from the brain only, arise our pleasures, joys, laughter and jests, as well as our sorrows, pains, griefs, and fears. Through it, in particular, we think, see, hear, and distinguish the ugly from the beautiful, the bad from the good, the pleasant from the unpleasant. . . . It is the same thing which makes us mad or delirious, inspires us with dread and fear, whether by night or by day, brings sleeplessness, inopportune mistakes, aimless anxieties, absentmindedness, and acts that are contrary to habit. These things that we suffer all come from the brain, when it is not healthy, but becomes abnormally hot, cold, moist, or dry, or suffers from any other unnatural affection to which it was not accustomed. Madness comes from its moistness.
>
> —HIPPOCRATES

The brain is the source of everything that we are. It is the source of everything that makes us human, humane, and unique. It is the source of our ability to speak, to write, to think, to create, to love, to laugh, to despair, and to hate.

Although Hippocrates, the "Father of Medicine," suspected the importance of the brain many years ago, we have not appreciated its nearly total dominance of our lives and selves until relatively recently. As our language indicates, we tend to speak and think as if we were controlled by something else. When we fall in love, we give someone our hearts, When we display our feelings, we wear our hearts on our sleeves. When we become very emotional, we spill our guts. When we make a joke, we are humorous. (The "humors" are the fluids of the body, like blood and bile.) When we are angry, we are pissed off. When we worry, our stomachs churn. In fact, we do all these things with our brains.

It was only natural that we were misled for centuries, and that most of us understand the importance of the brain only dimly. We all tend to believe what we can see or sense. We have all seen blood, urine, feces, and vomit. We hear our hearts beat and our stomachs growl. We all know that if our hearts stop beating, we will die. We know that while we are living, the heart pumps the fluid through our body that carries most of its nourishment. Therefore, the heart in particular has seemed to be the seat of our lives, our souls, our identities, and by implication our thoughts and feelings.

Only in very recent years have we realized that life resides in the brain. The heart, which seemed so important, is relatively insignificant. The heart is a simple mechanical pump made of muscle tissue. It can be stopped, as it is during open-heart surgery, and life can be sustained by a machine. Hearts can be transplanted from one person to another without causing an iota of change in their thoughts or feelings, except to the extent that the experience of illness and surgery affects them. Within the past several years, in fact, doctors have even used a totally artificial mechanical pump to replace diseased hearts. For many years, portions of the heart have been replaced with artificial parts, such as new valves.

To do any of these things with the brain is unthinkable. Its parts are irreplaceable. When a part is damaged or lost, as during a stroke or head injury, an important component of a cognitive function is damaged or lost forever. The person has difficulty talking, or seeing, or recognizing familiar faces. Although retraining, as through speech therapy, may help, the injury cannot be remedied by replacing the damaged bit of brain. Whole brains will probably never be transplanted. The operation is too difficult, because brain tissue is very sensitive and delicate, and because the brain has complex connections to too many different parts of the body. But even were whole brain transplants technically possible, they would be resisted on moral and ethical grounds, for to transplant a brain is to transplant a personality, an identity, perhaps a soul.

When a brain dies, as it usually does after about five to ten minutes if its blood supply is cut off, the essence of the person also dies. Sometimes the heart lives on without the brain, and these cases are the most tragic that families and physicians must deal with. "Brain death," evidenced by an absence of electrical activity in the brain (a "flat EEG" or electroencephalogram), means that the person has lost all of the abilities that make him human. Or, as we often say, he is "like a vegetable." Fortunately, heart death usually occurs simultaneously with, or soon after, brain death, and so such examples of the preeminence of the brain are not common.

What is this important organ really like? Why did we misunderstand it for so long?

It seems very remote to most of us. Few people have ever seen a human brain or realized that they were getting a glimpse of any of its parts. Thus the brain seems distant, ethereal, and cerebral. In fact, we can all see a bit of it, for the lining of the eyes is composed of an extension of the brain outside the skull. The back of the eye, or retina, consists of small nerve cells that begin within the brain and are part of it. (This is what a doctor is examining when he looks into your eyes with an ophthalmoscope.) Perhaps that is why we so often sense what people are really thinking or feeling by watching their eyes. But that is our only obvious contact with the brain, and most of us do not even suspect what we might be indirectly observing.

If we were to look at the human brain, as a few curious scientists and artists have done for centuries, we would not find it to be obviously impressive, nor would its workings be quickly apparent. Its most impressive aspect is its size. It looks like a large hunk of rather shapeless creamy-pinkish fat. Its surface is covered with furrows, but beneath these furrows it looks more or less the same throughout. The surface area is somewhat darker than the rest of the brain, and it has therefore come to be called "gray matter." But most of the brain is creamy in color, and it is called "white matter." For no apparent reason and in no obvious pattern, there are a few areas of gray matter embedded deep within the white matter. The brain is divided into two globular halves—the left and right hemispheres—which appear to be more or less symmetrical and are attached to one another by a thin strip of white matter called the "corpus callosum" (tough body). Both hemispheres are also attached to a thick, ropy structure, the spinal cord, which travels down the back encased in vertebrae and sends out small threads of nerve bundles that connect the brain with the rest of the body.

The brain itself is soft, delicate, and easily damaged. If you touch it too hard, it may bleed. It is encased in the thick, bony skull, making it difficult to reach and examine, and within the skull it is covered with a tough fibrous sac (the dura mater, or "hard mother") filled with a fluid in which it is suspended and cushioned, the cerebrospinal fluid. It is well protected, better protected than any other part of the body. Its designer, if it had one, concealed it well from hostile forces, in addition to concealing well its organization and function.

The appearance of the brain is very deceptive. If we try to see it as did the early medical explorers who were attempting to understand the nature and functions of various bodily organs, its most obvious features would appear to be its inaccessibility, its rather homogeneous texture and appearance, and its connections to many different parts of the body through the spinal cord. The other bodily organ that it seems to resemble most closely is the liver, for with the liver the brain shares a large size, a relatively homogeneous appearance, and a friable texture making it prone to bleed easily. It is quite unlike the heart, whose functions are relatively more obvious because its structure provides many clues to its purpose. The heart has four hollow chambers that are filled with blood and connected by large vessels to the rest of the body. One set of vessels carries blood back and forth between the lungs and the right side of the heart, while the other set of vessels carries blood back and forth to the rest of the body. In spite of these obvious clues, the function of the heart and the circulation of the blood were not discovered until the seventeenth century by William Harvey. Small wonder that the brain has begun to reveal its secrets to scientists only recently.

The single most important fact about the brain is very well disguised. Although all of this large mass of squishy, fatty tissue looks more or less the same, different parts are highly specialized. The brain has a complicated structure, and portions that are identical in appearance control our ability to perform very different mental and bodily functions. We use one part when we talk, another when we kick a football, and yet another when we survey the landscape with our eyes. Yet all these parts are connected to one another and interact with one another. During the course of the past century and a half, scientists have been using ingenious methods to map the localization of these various functions in the brain and to understand how it works.

The scientific era of brain research began in the nineteenth century. In its earliest phases, the scientific era depended heavily on "natural experiments"—the study of people who had suffered damage to their brains from stroke or head injury. The part of the brain that was accurately mapped the earliest was the language region, which is located in the left hemisphere. This story begins in 1837, when Marc Dax, a country doctor who had spent most of his life ministering to the ill rather than doing scientific research, presented a paper at a medical society meeting in Montpellier, France. The topic of the paper was aphasia, or loss of the ability to speak. Dax had noticed that in more than forty patients whom he had cared for, loss of ability to speak was associated with paralysis on the right side of the body and damage to the left hemisphere. He presented the rather striking conclusion that different parts of the brain might be specialized to perform different functions, and that in particular the ability to speak was located in the left hemisphere. This point of view has come to be called the "localization hypothesis."

Dax's conclusions did not arouse much interest in those attending the meeting, not to mention other doctors in France or the rest of the world. Most people continued to believe that we use our entire brain, acting as a unit, when we speak, write, move, or perceive. Only a German anatomist, Franz Gall, who founded the science of phrenology, had been a strong believer in the localization hypothesis. Because Gall also believed that the underlying anatomy and primacy of functions could be deduced by palpating bumps on the skull, a belief that was quickly found to be erroneous, the localization hypothesis tended to be considered quackery and pseudoscience. Only a few scientists continued to pursue it.

This situation changed dramatically in 1861, when a Parisian surgeon, Paul Broca, presented data to the Society of Anthropology in Paris about a patient whom he called "Tan." Tan was an old man who had suffered a stroke that left the right side of his body paralyzed and his speech so impaired that he was limited to saying only the word *Tan.* He was able to express himself to a small degree, however, by changing the intonation to convey different meanings. Tan eventually died, and Broca was therefore able to perform an autopsy to examine his brain. Although Broca examined only the external surface of the brain, he identified an area of damaged tissue in the back part of the third ridge of the frontal lobe on the left side, a region that has since come to be called "Broca's area." He presented this case, and later another one, to the Society of Anthropology.

Not everyone was willing to accept the implications of this finding, and during the next several years heated debate occurred between those brain scientists who hypothesized that brain functions were well localized and those who believed that they were primarily generalized. But by 1864, Broca was able to conclude that *"nous parlons avec l'hemisphere gauche"* ("we speak with the left half of our brains"). This side of the brain also controls motor function on the right side of the body and is opposite from the side of the dominant hand, the one that we use to write or throw a ball. He suspected that a reversal of this specialization could occur in left-handers, who might speak with their right hemispheres. (We now know that this is usually not true.)

Broca's work truly revolutionized the way we have come to think about the nature of the brain. It suggested two major ideas: cerebral specialization and cerebral dominance. Cerebral specialization implies that different parts of the brain perform different functions. Cerebral dominance suggests that the two halves of the brain, which appear to be nearly identical and symmetrical, are not mere duplications of one another, but may perform differing and perhaps complementary types of mental activities, with the left being more dominant in that it performs more complex or sophisticated functions, such as speech.

The next few years were full of feverish activity in the brain sciences, as clinicians and researchers began to explore the exciting idea that various regions of control could indeed be mapped in the brain. The story soon became even more interesting and more complicated. For example, the next step was the recognition that language functions were not single and simple. In 1876 Carl Wernicke, a German neurologist, presented data concerning patients who could speak fluently, although their speech made little sense, but who were unable to understand what others said to them. These patients had damage to a different part of the brain that was located farther back in a region that has come to be known as "Wernicke's area." These findings suggested that we use one part of our brain when we speak and yet another when we listen to others speak. Clearly, the mapping of brain specialization was going to require very fine detail.

The story of that mapping continues down to the present time and is summarized in later sections of this chapter. Beginning with the language center in the left hemisphere, scientists have moved to other regions of the brain and charted their functions in a detail that would make Gall and his fellow phrenologists envious. Unlike Gall's charts, which were based on theories and faulty evidence, the modern charts of brain function are based on a century of carefully accumulated and critically scrutinized data.

Before Continuing: A Caveat

The growth of our understanding about how the brain works is perhaps the most exciting story in the history of science. On the other hand, anyone who tries to absorb all the knowledge that has accumulated by the mid-1980s may find the task nearly overwhelming, particularly if one begins without any background in chemistry or biological sciences. The neurosciences are notoriously difficult for all beginning students for several different reasons.

First of all, the terminology used to describe the structure of the brain is not easy to learn. It has been slowly accumulating for centuries, and without some knowledge of how it developed, it is almost impossible to remember much of it. The earliest terminology derived from Latin and Greek, the language of science and scholarship until relatively recently. This terminology tends to describe the shape and appearance of structures, usually without much relation to their function or location. Thus we have terms like *amygdala* (almond), *mammillary bodies* (breastlike structures), *hippocampus* (sea horse), *fornix* (arch), *corpus callosum* (tough body), and even *substantia innominata* (unnamed substance). Some of these structures have been renamed over the years so that terminology could become simplified, but many scientists have been reluctant to abandon the old names. Thus the large fold or fissure separating the temporal lobe from the rest of the brain is called both the "Sylvian fissure" and the "lateral fissure." Learning even a smattering of brain anatomy, enough to understand what the structures are and how they work, involves learning a large number of terms that are both arbitrary and inconsistent. In a sense, learning the vocabulary of the brain is like learning a foreign language.

A second factor that makes it difficult to gain a firm hold on how the brain works is the fact that it is a very complicated three-dimensional structure. Its superficial appearance of homogeneity and simplicity is incredibly deceptive. The little patches of gray matter scattered within the brain and given silly names such as "almond" or "breast" are connected to one another and to the rest of the brain. These patches of gray matter are information centers that communicate with one another and control our behavior and feelings. In other words, there are in fact many different structures or systems within the brain. Their connections to one another are quite complicated and difficult to remember. Indeed, many are not yet known; this is one of the many exciting frontiers of research within the neurosciences. Because these different functional and anatomical systems are three-dimensional, stretching from the front of the brain to the back and from one side to the other, as well as being nested inside one another, it is difficult for most people to develop a clear mental image of the structure of the brain, even with the assistance of good illustrations.

A third factor complicating our understanding of the brain is that there is no accurate model or metaphor to describe how it works. For the atom we have the solar system. For DNA we have the double helix. Models have, of course, been proposed for the brain. Perhaps the commonest is the computer, which stores and retrieves information with astonishing efficiency and can be programmed to use this stored information to perform complex tasks like playing chess. But the human brain is different from a computer in many ways that make the computer model an oversimplification. The human brain differs from a computer in that it is smarter even though it is less efficient. For example, it can be creative and modify what it is doing if things are not working, while a computer simply "tilts." When confronted with a new problem, the computer refuses to run, fails to recognize the problem, gives the wrong solution, and is infuriatingly inflexible, as all of us who must communicate with the computers of insurance agencies or businesses (or even those residing in our homes) know only too well. The human brain can often recognize a problem and correct it instantly. Computers can think only digitally or incrementally. The information that they store is usually in 1-0 (or yes-no, present-absent) form. On the other hand, the human brain can think and perceive in infinitely fine shades of meaning. The human brain can forget, while the computer can only remember. Thus, although the computer provides a useful model for some aspects of mental functioning, particularly the way information is stored and retrieved, it cannot explain everything. In fact, the human brain is probably too complex to lend itself to any single metaphor.

An alternate metaphor that may be helpful, however, is to think of the brain as a very large network of different communication centers that can flash on and off and send messages to one another through electrical impulses. The brain contains many different specialized information centers scattered throughout its three-dimensional space. These highly specialized areas of gray matter are centers or way stations that contain the ability to remember, to formulate decisions, and to issue commands. Different areas of gray matter are specialized in different functions, such as moving, seeing, touching, listening, thinking, or modulating physical functions such as eating or sleeping. Often these areas are redundant—that is, several areas can perform the same function. Thus, when one communication center is knocked out through disease, another may be able to take over in its place.

These specialized areas of gray matter are connected to one another through fibers that are like wires; these fiber tracts are the material that we see in the brain as white matter. When communication between the centers in the brain breaks down, it may be due either to direct damage to a center of gray matter or to damage to the wiring between the centers. Often the connections between centers are also redundant, however, so that when damage occurs, messages can be sent through alternate connections. Thus the brain has an amazing adaptive capacity that is sometimes referred to as "plasticity." When the brain is working at its usual busy level of performance, it can be thought of as a three-dimensional layout of electrical switchboards in which many different areas are receiving messages, "lighting up," and sending messages back in response.

The sections that follow describe the structural and functional organization of the brain. You have been forewarned that it will be dense with dull and arbitrary terminology. Because dividing things into smaller parts is an easy way for us to learn and remember, the following sections divide the brain into various rather traditional divisions. Be forewarned in this regard as well: These divisions are both arbitrary and oversimplified, since the essence of the brain is not so much its parts as it is the connections between the parts.

How Is the Brain Constructed?

LARGE-SCALE STRUCTURES

To understand how the brain works, we must look at it at different levels. Conceptualizing the brain at any one level is purely arbitrary, since a complete understanding of how the brain works must synthesize all these levels. Nevertheless, one must begin somewhere, and we will begin by looking first at the large-scale structure of the brain, otherwise known as its gross anatomy. Among the neurosciences, this particular branch is called "neuroanatomy." As we grow in our understanding of the localization of mental and emotional functions within the brain, we may also begin to speak of "psychoanatomy."

Studying the gross anatomy of the brain involves looking at structures one can see with the naked eye. When one begins to look at smaller structures that one can see only with a microscope, such as nerve cells and fibers, then one is learning about the neurohistology or neuropathology of the brain. Finally, since most of the activity of the brain involves communication between cells and fibers by means of electrical impulses set off by chemical messengers, one learns about the functioning of the brain at the electrical level through the study of neurophysiology and at the molecular level through the study of neurochemistry. We shall begin, however, by looking at the brain as the first scientists did, before the dawn of modern physiology and chemistry.

If one were to remove a brain from the skull, it would appear in side view just as it does in figure 1. Its surface is highly convoluted and folded, so that a relatively large surface can be crowded into a relatively small space. The brain of an average man weighs about three pounds; women's brains are somewhat smaller. Brain size is closely related to head size, but has no relationship to intelligence. The ridges of the brain are called "gyri" (singular: gyrus); the wrinkles between them are called "sulci" (singular: sulcus) or "fissures."

Figure 2 shows some of the parts into which the brain is traditionally divided. It is useful to think of the brain as containing six or seven component parts.

The largest and most advanced part consists of the left and right cerebral hemispheres, which appear more or less symmetrical and identical to the untutored naked eye. They are covered with a layer of gray matter called the "cerebral cortex," or "bark" of the brain. Indeed, when the brain is cut into sections, as shown in figure 4, it does appear somewhat like a tree trunk with dark bark on the outside and lighter material inside. The light material is the white matter, or wiring, that connects various regions of the cortex to other brain centers.

Each of the cerebral hemispheres has traditionally been divided into four "lobes," which are named after the bones of the skull that surround them: frontal, parietal, occipital, and temporal. These lobes are demarcated by fissures, or sulci, that are often difficult for the

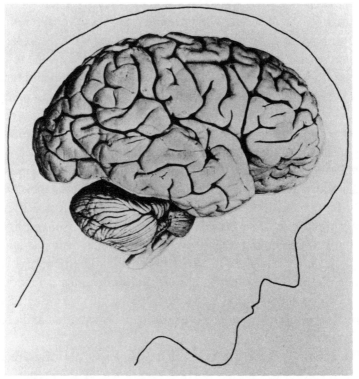

Fig. 1. The human brain, as seen from the right side.

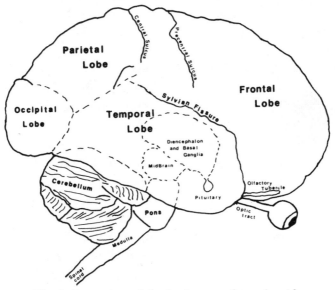

Fig. 2. Structures of the brain, seen from the side.

untrained eye to observe. They are also said to have different functions, but any brief summary of their functions is likely to be oversimplified and is best regarded as such. The frontal lobe is the largest and least understood, beginning at the front of the brain and reaching back to the central sulcus. The area between the central and precentral sulci helps control body movements and is called the "motor area," while the remainder of the frontal lobe probably modulates various aspects of thinking, feeling, imagining, and making decisions. The parietal lobe is the region behind the central sulcus. Part of it is called the "somatosensory area," since it receives information about various bodily sensations; the parietal lobe also modulates such activities as spatial orientation. The occipital lobe receives and sends out visual information. The boundaries between the parietal, occipital, and temporal lobes are rather blurry to the naked eye. The temporal lobe is perhaps the most conspicuous lobe of the brain since it juts out and forward from the rest and is demarcated by the very deep Sylvian fissure. The temporal lobe receives auditory information and controls memory and language.

The activities these two cerebral hemispheres perform are sometimes referred to as "higher cortical functions." The cerebral hemispheres are much larger and more convoluted in human beings than in any other animals. Further, they contain the capacity for some functions that no other animals possess, such as the ability to speak, read, or write in a highly developed language. Consequently, many neuroscientists believe that the cerebral hemispheres are the part of the brain that makes us uniquely human.

The cerebral hemispheres are sometimes referred to as the "telencephalon," or "endbrain," since they are the most highly developed of the brain structures. The next sets of structures within the brain are the diencephalon, or "betweenbrain," and the basal ganglia, or "lower nerve knots." These structures cannot be seen from the outside of the brain, for they are embedded deep within it. They are shown in dotted lines in figure 2 and can be seen in more detail in subsequent figures. These structures consist of small masses of gray matter made up of the cell bodies of neurons. They serve as relay stations between lower brain centers and the higher cortical centers. The most important structures in the diencephalon are the thalamus (or "marriage bed") and the hypothalamus (below the thalamus). The thalamus is an important meeting place that joins many brain centers to one another and serves as a modulator of movement, sensation, emotions, and behavior, while the hypothalamus regulates hormonal function. The basal ganglia serve as regulators of body movements.

The midbrain, pons (bridge), and medulla (marrow) comprise three more parts of the brain and are sometimes grouped together and called the "brainstem." This portion of the brain is the most primitive and is primarily concerned with survival capacities. It regulates the activity of the heart, respiration, and other vital functions. In addition, it receives information from the remainder of the body through the spinal cord and the cranial nerves. (The cranial nerves are twelve different nerve bundles located primarily in the brainstem that send information to and from the head and neck; the olfactory nerve to the nose and the optic nerve to the eye are examples of these cranial nerves.) The cerebellum is sometimes considered a part of the midbrain and sometimes treated as a separate structure. It is a relatively large and intensely foliated structure that serves as a major modulator of movement, working together with motor regions of the cortex as well as the basal ganglia.

LOOKING INSIDE THE BRAIN

In order to reconstruct the brain in its full three-dimensional complexity, we have to cut it in different ways and see what we then discover. Figure 3 shows what one sees when one splits the brain down the middle, dividing it into two separate hemispheres and cutting away the cerebellum and brainstem. Although these latter structures are very important in overall bodily functions, they have little relevance to the higher functions that are disturbed during mental illness, and therefore are outside the scope of this book.

In side view we again see that a large part of the brain is composed of the mysterious frontal lobe. A large, arching frontal gyrus is seen jutting forward just above the eyeball (the straight gyrus) and sweeping around the front of the brain and over its top (e.g., the superior frontal gyrus). Beneath this frontal gyrus is another large ridge of cortex, the cingulate (girdling) gyrus. This gyrus, while technically within the frontal lobe, is in fact part of yet another brain system that appears in both the frontal and temporal lobes and is also connected to a variety of gray-matter centers that are deep inside the brain. This

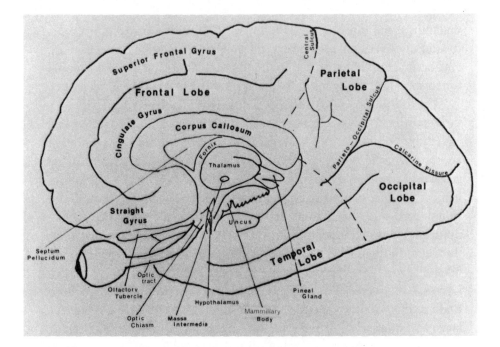

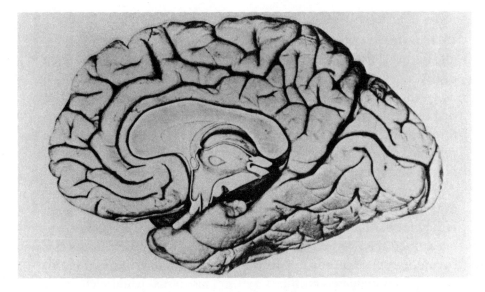

Fig. 3. The human brain, sectioned down the middle.

system, which is an important modulator of emotions and may be one of the systems that breaks down during mental illness, is called the "limbic," or "border," system. The cortical part of this system that we see in figure 2 consists of the cingulate gyrus, which arches back around the corpus callosum, connects with the parahippocampal gyrus in the temporal lobe, and curves under to form the uncus (or hook). Subcortical portions of the limbic system that we can also see from this midline view include the septal region near the septum pellucidum (or translucent divider), the fornix, and the mammillary bodies. As we saw from the side view, from the midline view we can also see sections of the parietal, occipital, and temporal lobes. Sometimes these are neatly demarcated by familiar sulci, such as the central sulcus or parie-to-occipital sulcus, while in other instances the margins are purely arbitrary when viewed with the naked eye. We shall see later that these regions do differ from one another at the smaller histological level because they contain different types of nerve cells organized in different types of layers.

When we cut the brain down the middle, we cut through a number of important fiber tracts that provide communication between the two hemispheres. The largest of these fiber tracts is the corpus callosum. Until only ten to twenty years ago, many scientists thought that the corpus callosum had no important function. Medical students were sometimes taught that it served as a buttress to keep the hemispheres from sagging. However, the recent work of brain scientists such as Norman Geschwind and Roger Sperry has demonstrated that this portion of the brain wires the two halves of the brain together and is continually busy transferring messages from one side to the other in order to call on various specialized functions or abilities.

In the side view shown in figure 3, several other structures have been cut in two. The pineal gland, once thought to be a "third eye" and now thought to partially regulate the sleep-wake cycle, resides just below the posterior end of the corpus callosum. The mammillary bodies are paired, and one of them has been cut away. These small but important structures are part of the brain system that permits us to learn and remember. The area to their right with a jagged edge would connect to the brainstem had not this structure been cut away to reveal the underlying temporal lobe. Toward the front, the two optic tracts, which carry fibers from the nerve cells lining the back of the eyeball, jut out to either side. These tracts cross, as do many in the brain, and their place of crossing is called the "optic chiasm," which has also been cut away. Just above the optic tract one sees the olfactory tubercle, a cranial nerve collecting information about how things smell. In the middle of all these structures, one sees a thalamus, that important "marriage bed" or relay station that we will soon learn about in more detail. There are two thalami, one on each side of the brain, and they are usually fused in the midline by the massa intermedia. Arching above the thalamus is the fornix, part of the limbic system, while below it are the structures of the hypothalamus, too small to be seen at this anatomic level.

Our third perspective on the three-dimensional structure of the brain comes from cutting through it in various planes. Figure 4 shows what one may see in one such cut. The actual brain structures appear in figure 4A, while the angle of the cut and a diagrammatic representation appear in figure 4B. This cut shows most clearly the barklike quality of the cerebral cortex. It also shows vividly that one indeed finds many peculiar islands of gray matter buried deeply inside the cortex. In subsequent figures we will examine in more detail the complex three-dimensional relationship of these subcortical structures and systems.

In looking at this slice of brain, we must regard it with the same puzzlement as did the early explorers of brain anatomy. We see the by now rather familiar but also rather arbitrary division of the brain into the frontal, temporal, and occipital lobes. Only a small portion of the parietal lobe, which typically occurs higher up, is seen on this section. The cingulate gyrus and the hippocampus reappear, although it is no longer obvious that they are connected to one another.

In this cut, one can perhaps see best that the corpus callosum does contain fibers joining the two hemispheres. Tiny hollow areas appear, labeled in this cut as the frontal and temporal horns of the lateral ventricles. These are portions of the brain containing cerebrospinal fluid and also having a complicated shape that will be shown in more detail in a later figure. The frontal horns are bounded on either side by the caudate (taillike) nuclei, which are also part of the basal ganglia, as are the claustrum (cloister) and the putamen (stone). Because of their shape, they have sometimes been called the "lenticular" (lenslike) nuclei and the "corpus striatum" (striped body). The large

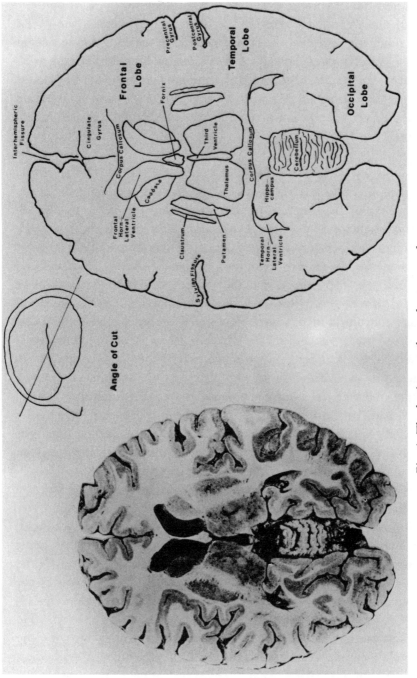

Fig. 4. The brain, cut through at an angle.

oval thalami reappear in the midline with the tiny, slitlike third ventricle, also full of cerebrospinal fluid, lying between them.

If one were to cut through the brain at lower levels, one would see other structures and substantially more of the cerebellum; a cut at higher levels would show more of the parietal lobe. Most of the gross structure of the brain has been discovered in the past by such laborious cutting at various levels, with considerable effort and imagination being used to determine what structures were actually related to one another.

THE LIMBIC SYSTEM

Among these varied systems of gray matter buried deep inside the brain, the limbic system is perhaps of greatest interest to psychiatry. As we shall see in a subsequent section, early in this century Brodmann, a member of Kraepelin's Department of Psychiatry in Munich, studied the appearance of different types of brain cells under the microscope. He noticed that the organization of cell structures in some parts of the cortex, particularly the cingulate gyrus, appeared much more primitive. Hence this part of the brain came to be called "paleocortex," or "old cortex," in contrast to the more highly developed cortex of other regions ("neocortex," or "new cortex"). Because this part of the cortex was also close to, and appeared to be connected with, the olfactory tubercle, it was also called the "rhinencephalon," or "nose brain," and thought to be concerned primarily with the sense of smell. The term *limbic lobe* (bordering lobe) was introduced by Broca in order to refer to those cortical regions seen on midline section that border the corpus callosum.

Except for simple anatomical descriptions, the nature and function of the limbic system were shrouded in mystery until relatively recently. In 1937, James Papez, a professor at Cornell Medical School, dramatically changed the way brain scientists perceived the limbic system when he introduced the idea of the "Papez circuit." While other brain scientists had been busy determining which parts of the brain are used to move our limbs or to hear or to see, Papez asked, "What part of the brain is used to feel and to regulate emotion?" He speculated that the structures involved in this process included the cingulate gyrus, the hippocampus, the fornix, the mammillary bodies, and parts of the thalamus. Papez believed that experiences perceived through more sophisticated parts of the brain were funneled to the more primitive and deeper structures by the cingulate gyrus and the hippocampus. These in turn sent messages by way of the fornix to the mammillary bodies of the hypothalamus, which then communicated back to the thalamus, which in turn communicated back to the cingulate gyrus.

Thus, Papez thought of emotional experience and expression as a reverberating circuit: Within this circuit, emotion tended to build up in the hippocampal area, while the cingulate gyrus was responsible for emotional awareness. The original Papez circuit, shown in figure 5, has now been substantially enlarged, amplified, and revised. Indeed, we are still in the process of learning all the various connections and functions of the limbic system.

A more modern, but still oversimplified and incomplete, view of

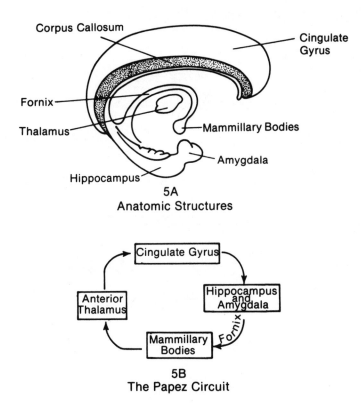

5A
Anatomic Structures

5B
The Papez Circuit

Fig. 5. The limbic system as conceptualized by Papez.

the limbic system is portrayed in figure 6 in somewhat schematic fashion. Figure 6A shows the major structures that are considered to be part of the limbic system or closely related to it. Some of these, such as the frontal lobe, are not part of the limbic system as narrowly defined, but are connected with it in important ways. Within figure 6A we note several new anatomic structures that were not described as part of the original limbic system. In particular, these include the tiny but important septal nuclei and the habenular nucleus.

Some of the various connections of the limbic system and the interrelationship between its parts are shown in figure 6B. The origi-

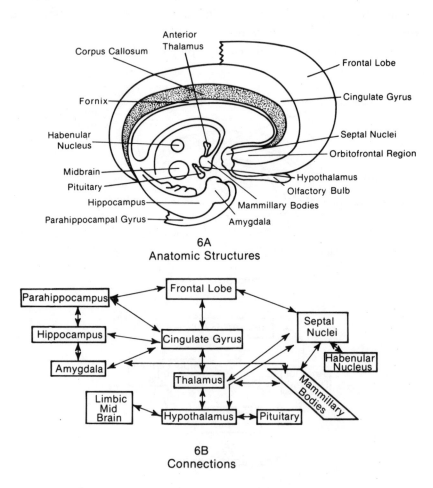

6A
Anatomic Structures

6B
Connections

Fig. 6. **The modern limbic system.**

nal Papez circuit has clearly become much more complicated. Information from the external environment is collected through the parahippocampus of the temporal lobe, the frontal lobe and cingulate gyrus, and the olfactory bulb. The thalamus and septal nuclei serve as major way stations that pass information on from other major structures, such as the mammillary bodies, hypothalamus, amygdala, or hippocampus. Circuits are also available for many of these structures to communicate back to one another. Some of these structures within the limbic system—such as the septal nuclei, mammillary bodies, amygdala, and hippocampus—have been shown to be important receivers and regulators of information, since damage to these structures produces loss of the ability to learn new information and retain it in long-term memory. Other structures, such as the hypothalamus and pituitary, are regulators of hormonal functioning, governing activities such as thirst, sex drive, and appetite. Still other structures—such as the cingulate gyrus and frontal lobe—are known to be involved in the ability to think creatively and make decisions, and they also modulate the ability to start and stop various behaviors. Thus the components and connections of the limbic system contain most of the elements that define individual personality, cognitive style, and patterns of behavior.

Although the original hypothesis of Papez has been modified, many brain scientists retain his basic belief that the key to understanding many aspects of mental illness may lie within the limbic system and its connections. This may be the part of the brain that has been somehow "broken" in at least some of those patients suffering from the schizophrenias or the affective disorders. No specific defect in the limbic system has been uncovered as yet, but a clustering of evidence from the study of brain chemistry and the effects of drugs contains many tantalizing hints.

THE BASAL GANGLIA

Many of the structures of the limbic system, such as the fornix or mammillary bodies, are nested deep inside the brain. On either side of these midline structures, we find another set of gray-matter structures that also serve as important way stations: the basal ganglia (lower nerve knots). In simplified form, the limbic system is thought of as modulating emotions, memory, and perhaps aspects of attention, while the basal ganglia are considered to be modulators of movement and integrators of sensory information. We saw some important parts of the basal ganglia in cross-section in figures 4A and 4B, the caudate and putamen.

Although structures modulating movement or integrating sensation might, at first thought, seem to have little to do with the study of mental illness, in fact knowledge of the basal ganglia is important for several reasons. First, they are related neurochemically to the limbic system. As we shall see shortly, messages are carried through the brain by means of a variety of chemical substances referred to as "neurotransmitters." Different portions of the brain use different kinds of neurotransmitters. The basal ganglia share with the limbic system a particular neurotransmitter, dopamine, that is considered to be important in the development of schizophrenia. Consequently, some neuroscientists believe that the study of the basal ganglia may improve our understanding of schizophrenia, which may even be related to recognized diseases of the basal ganglia.

Second, we already know quite a bit about the basal ganglia, which tend to be selectively damaged in various types of disease. For example, Huntington's chorea, a hereditary illness with a clearly defined pattern of genetic transmission (autosomal dominance), is characterized by a "broken" caudate nucleus. Another well-recognized disease, Parkinson's disease, results from the death of nerve cells in the substantia nigra (black substance), a gray-matter center that is part of the basal ganglia but is located in the midbrain. Finally, both of these diseases of the basal ganglia have symptoms similar to those noticed in the common major mental illnesses, such as schizophrenia and affective disorders. Patients with Huntington's chorea often develop depression or delusional thinking. Patients with Parkinson's disease have changes in the expression of affect and loss of volition similar to those noted in schizophrenia.

Like the limbic system, the basal ganglia have a complex three-dimensional shape involving connections between different way stations of gray matter. The components are shown in figure 7. The large caudate nucleus begins deep inside the frontal lobe near the midline and arches back to form a C-shaped structure that ends on either side deep inside the temporal lobe. The caudate is connected to the amygdala, which is part of the limbic system.

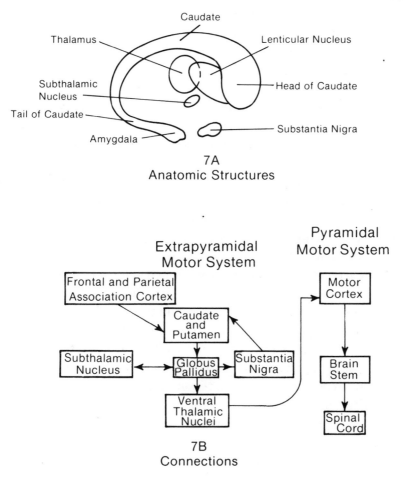

7A
Anatomic Structures

7B
Connections

Fig. 7. **Basal ganglia.**

Lateral to the caudate one finds the lenticular nucleus. This is composed of two different types of gray matter. On the inside one finds the globus pallidus (pale globe), which is a somewhat lighter mass of gray matter than its adjacent neighbor, the putamen. That important marriage chamber, the thalamus, contains significant connections to these knots of gray matter and is sometimes considered part of the basal ganglia. It lies slightly farther back and inside the lenticular nucleus. The relationship of these structures is best seen cross-sectionally in figure 4. In that figure, one also notices the claustrum, a gray-matter mass that appears to be related to the basal ganglia physically but whose function has as yet not been discovered.

These various structures are connected to the subthalamic nucleus in the diencephalon and to the substantia nigra in the midbrain. Because these structures have a striped appearance when cut through, they are called the "striatum" (striped area). Sometimes neuroscientists distinguish between the neostriatum or "new striatum" (caudate and putamen) and the paleostriatum or "old striatum" (globus pallidus) because the latter contains different types of cells that are clearly more primitive.

The connections of the basal ganglia and their relationship to the motor system are shown in figure 7B. As that figure shows, there are really two major motor systems within the brain. The most sophisticated system, shown on the right of the diagram, is sometimes called the "pyramidal system" because its fiber tracts have a pyramidlike shape on cut section. This system sends a chain of command from the motor cortex down through the brainstem to the spinal cord and on out to the muscles of the body, with some modulating input from the thalamus. The basal ganglia lie within the second, more primitive motor system, sometimes referred to as the "extrapyramidal system" since it lies outside or separate from the pyramidal system. Within this system the chain of command runs from certain regions within the frontal and parietal cortex, which specialize in integrating information from the outside world (sometimes referred to as "association areas") down through the caudate and putamen to the globus pallidus and on to the thalamus. Feedback loops occur, however, in the globus pallidus and the subthalamic nucleus, as well as between the globus pallidus, substantia nigra, and caudate and putamen. Through the thalamus, the extrapyramidal system also "talks back" to the motor cortex.

The basal ganglia, or extrapyramidal system, serves as a modulating system for motor function. When portions of it are damaged, various kinds of abnormalities can be noticed. For example, damage to the caudate produces peculiar writhing and twitching movements, in addition to many other defects. Damage to the substantia nigra produces the symptoms of Parkinson's disease, such as tremulousness, rigidity, and a decrease in spontaneous movement sometimes referred to as "akinesia."

THE VENTRICULAR SYSTEM

The ventricular system is the final anatomic structure that we must examine. It, too, has a complicated three-dimensional shape, but its structure and function are relatively simple. The ventricular system consists of four fluid-filled cavities buried deep within the brain. Its appearance is portrayed in figure 8. There are two lateral ventricles, one within each hemisphere. Each of the lateral ventricles has projections into the frontal lobe, the occipital lobe, and the temporal lobe. The frontal and temporal horns of the lateral ventricles can also be seen on the cross-sectional cut of the brain shown in figure 4. These two lateral ventricles are connected to the much smaller midline third ventricle, which is surrounded on either side by the two thalami. The third ventricle stretches down and is connected to an even smaller fourth ventricle, which then flows into a fluid-filled column that runs through the center of the spinal cord. The ventricular system is filled with a watery fluid—the cerebrospinal fluid (CSF).

For centuries, people speculated that the ventricles might be the seat of the soul, no doubt in part because of their inaccessible location and perhaps because they are relatively conspicuous or obvious structures within the brain. In fact, however, the ventricular system plays a very minor role in brain function. The principal known purposes of

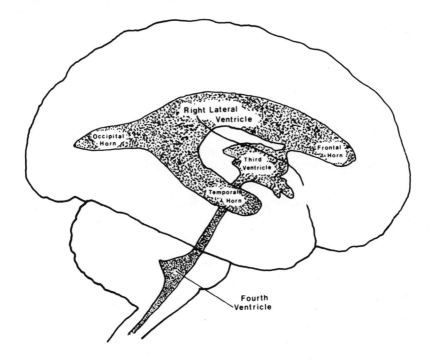

Fig. 8. The ventricular system.

the cerebrospinal fluid, which also bathes the outer surface of the brain, are to nourish and cushion it.

Nevertheless, the ventricular system is of interest to neuroscientists for several reasons. First of all, when brain cells are damaged or die, the substance of the brain grows smaller and the ventricles enlarge to fill the empty space within the skull; thus, ventricular enlargement provides a useful index of brain atrophy or shrinkage. A second reason that neuroscientists pay attention to the ventricular system is that the ventricles are major landmarks that can be seen very clearly using computerized tomographic brain scanning, a new X-ray technique developed in the 1970s. Ventricular enlargement has been noted in patients suffering from both dementia and schizophrenia, as will be discussed in more detail in chapter 7.

What Is the Functional Organization of the Brain?

In order to understand the brain, one must know its anatomy, but knowing anatomy is not enough. One also needs to know how the various parts of the brain are related to one another in order to perform various functions or tasks. What are some of these functional systems? Where are they located in the brain, and how do they work?

THE MOTOR SYSTEM

After Broca discovered the localization of speech in the posterior frontal area, another major finding quickly followed. Gustav Fritsch and Eduard Hitzig observed that electrical stimulation of the cortex in front of the central sulcus produced movement in dogs. As they continued their exploration, they also noticed that stimulating different portions of this "motor strip," as it has come to be called, led to movements of different parts of the body. For example, stimulation toward the top caused movements of the legs, while stimulation farther down, particularly in the area close to Broca's area and the temporal lobe, caused movements of the face, mouth, or tongue. The localization hypothesis received new and powerful support through their work. Otfried Furster described the motor cortex in much finer detail through surgical lesions in dogs. His findings were subsequently extended in the 1940s and 1950s through the research of Wilder Penfield, who mapped motor input to the various parts of the body by studying the effects of electrical stimulation on human beings during brain surgery for epilepsy. Since the patients were awake at the time, he was able to use their verbal reports to extend our knowledge of localization of function.

Penfield's detailed charting of the relationship between parts of the cortex and specific muscle groups is often called the "motor homunculus," which appears in figure 9. As that figure indicates, some parts of the body receive very little cortical input, while others receive a great deal. Only a tiny part of the brain is concerned with controlling the movements of our legs and arms, but our hands and faces, so important in supremely human activities such as playing the violin or talking, are controlled through very large portions of the motor cortex. Furthermore, motor control is highly lateralized: The left side of the brain governs the right side of the body, while the right brain governs the left side. No one knows why the brain is organized in this crossed pattern, which occurs in other systems besides the motor

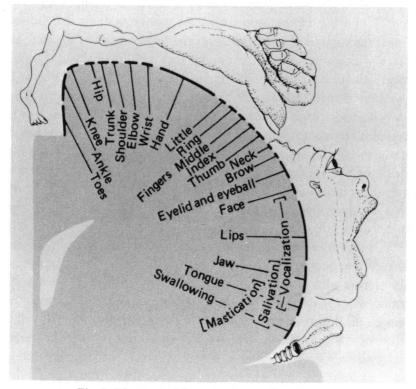

Fig. 9. The "motor homunculus" (after Penfield).

system. The crossing results from an actual physical crossing of nerve fibers in the brainstem.

Messages from the cortex reach our mouths, arms, and legs with the assistance of considerable modulation. After all, a command center is of little value if it does not receive information about whether its commands are being followed properly or whether there are factors in the outside world that prevent the commands from being carried out. Thus the motor system receives messages back from the body through information gathered by the eyes, the sense of touch, and many other sensory systems. As we have already seen, the basal ganglia also interact with the motor cortex and serve as modulators of it, as does the cerebellum.

THE SENSORY SYSTEM

The sensory system is composed of many systems widely distributed throughout the brain. Physical sensations are localized in a region called the "somatosensory area," located just behind the motor strip. While the motor strip forms the rear border of the frontal cortex, the somatosensory area forms the front border of the parietal cortex, which is devoted to integrating sensory information of various types. This area is constructed so that it is almost perfectly parallel with the motor strip in terms of the parts of the body that it controls. The somatosensory cortex receiving sensations from the arms and legs is adjacent to the motor strip that sends commands for movement to the arms and legs. Sensations from the face are received farther down the side of the brain in the sensory cortex and adjacent to the motor cortex controlling facial movement. Like the motor fibers, the sensory fibers are crossed, so that the left side of the brain feels what is happening on the right side of the body and vice versa.

This sensory area collects information about various bodily sensations, such as heat, cold, pain, and pressure or touch. The information sent to this part of the brain is collected by special receptor cells located all over the body. These receptors are designed to measure changes in things such as temperature or pressure to the skin. The information they collect is sent on to the thalamus by way of the spinal cord, and then on to the somatosensory cortex. Such information is collected with lightninglike speed and relayed quickly throughout the brain. For example, when your motor cortex commands your leg to move, sensory receptors in the foot quickly send back information to the brain indicating that your leg has moved and that your foot has indeed touched the ground. If it turns out that your foot has not touched the ground as expected (as when inadvertently stepping off a curb), messages sent to the basal ganglia and cerebellum permit these modulators of movement to tell your body how to readjust and regain its balance without causing you to fall or injure yourself.

The auditory and visual systems are additional major components of the sensory system. The visual system begins by collecting information in two highly specialized sensory receptors, our two eyes. A network of nerve cells—the retina (net)—lines the back of the eyeball. As they leave the eye, fibers from these photoreceptors are collected into a neat bundle called the "optic nerve." Optic-nerve fibers cross only partially and then pass into the substance of the brain, forming the optic tracts that send information to the visual cortex located in the very back of the brain in the occipital lobes. Like all other sensory systems providing input to the cortex, these nerves must make a stop in the thalamus, which probably serves as a filter to decide which among the various kinds of sensory messages it is receiving should be given higher priority and should be relayed on to the visual cortex for reconstruction.

Back in the visual cortex of the occipital lobes, the images seen by the eyes are reconstructed into understandable visual images, and then information is sent on to whatever part of the brain needs it. If you are concerned at the moment with hitting a tennis ball with a racket, then visual information about the location of the ball (and of your opponent) is sent on to the motor system so that you can move your body appropriately. On the other hand, if you are reading a book, the images of the letters on the page are sent on to the language system (about which more will follow later) in the temporal, parietal, and frontal lobes for decoding and reaction.

The auditory system follows a similar pattern. Like the eyes, the ears contain specialized receptors designed to collect information about the sounds that surround us. Information from these receptors passes into the brain through the left and right acoustic nerves, which send half of their fibers to the opposite hemisphere by way of the corpus callosum, as well as half to the same side (after making the usual first stop in the thalamus). The fibers passing from the left ear to the right hemisphere tend to send a more powerful signal, however, leading to what is sometimes called a "left-ear advantage." The auditory cortex in the temporal lobe interprets these signals and recognizes them as familiar melodies, familiar words, or signals of danger such as a honking horn. Depending on what we have heard, further information is sent on to the motor system so that we can move our bodies in a dance, or to the language system so that we can answer the question we have been asked.

THE LANGUAGE SYSTEM

The language system is unique to the human mind. Other primates, such as the chimpanzee, have brains that are very similar to that of man, and their chromosomes, which contain the genetic code that dictates the organization of their bodies, are nearly identical to human chromosomes. Very minute differences between primate and human chromosomes and brains lead to an enormous difference in the kinds of existences they are able to achieve. If one is asked "What is man?" one would have to reply that man's chief difference from the rest of the animal world rests in his ability to speak in a highly refined and complicated language. From this ability, which is programmed only in the human brain in intricate detail, evolves the capacity to express thoughts and feelings to other people, to produce literature, to write music, to preserve historical records, to articulate religious beliefs, to create mathematical systems, and to design and record scientific experiments.

The language system is located almost totally in the left hemisphere in most people. (About one-third of left-handers, however, either use their right hemisphere for language or use both hemispheres.) A diagram of the language system appears in figure 10. The components of the language system include Broca's area in the frontal lobe, the auditory cortex and Wernicke's area in the temporal lobe, the angular gyrus in the parietal lobe, and the visual area in the occipital lobe. These various areas are specialized regions connected to one another by nerve-fiber tracts. Damage to any particular center or to the connecting fiber tracts leads to different kinds of language abnormalities, and it is through the study of these various abnormalities that the language system has been mapped over the years. Other brain systems, such as the motor or sensory systems, also exist in the

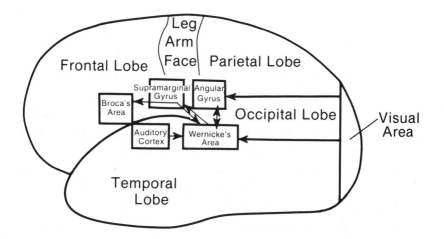

Fig. 10. The language system (after Damasio).

lower animals, and so it has been possible to study them through animal experiments. The language system, however, can be studied only through "natural experiments" such as stroke or head injury, since it exists only in man. The various disorders that occur when different parts of the language system are damaged are called the "aphasias."

Our understanding of how the language system works has been advanced greatly through the work of Norman Geschwind and his colleagues in Boston. According to Geschwind's model, the brain contains several different specialized centers governing language function. Broca's area is the part of the brain that contains information about details of grammar and provides the information permitting people to organize words into fluent speech. Damage to Broca's area leads to difficulty in speaking fluently and in particular to great difficulty in using the "little words" that carry a large burden of grammatical meaning—prepositions like *in* and *on,* pronouns like *he* and *it,* conjunctions like *and* and *or.* The angular gyrus is the language storehouse that contains the information that permits us to recognize language when it is presented in visual form. Wernicke's area is an analogous storage center programmed to permit us to recognize information presented in auditory form. When we hear speech, it is forwarded from the auditory cortex to Wernicke's area, where it is understood or comprehended.

Very likely, Wernicke's area serves as a storehouse of acoustical templates that permit us to recognize spoken words and attach meanings to them. Sometimes it is referred to as an "association area" because it contains the meanings that are associated with sounds. The sound *sweet* evokes associations of sugary taste or emotional gentleness. The sound *silent* suggests stillness and peace. When we hear a phrase such as "When to the sessions of sweet silent thought," each word is rapidly processed and coded with a meaning in Wernicke's area, and the phrase is then "understood." (No doubt the linguistic richness of great writers is due to an especially well-developed Wernicke's area!) If the speech that is heard calls for a reply, then a message is forwarded on to Broca's area so that a reply can be encoded in grammatical speech and then spoken.

Our ability to read begins with input to the visual cortex, which forwards images to the angular gyrus, where they are recognized and understood. Damage to the angular gyrus leads to loss of the ability to read and write, the two modes of language that are mediated visually. Damage to Wernicke's area leaves a person with the ability to speak without the ability to comprehend the meaning of speech. People with this form of damage, called "Wernicke's aphasia," produce fluent meaningless speech that is sometimes described as "word salad" or "jargon aphasia." Damage to the white-matter tracts connecting these speech centers can cause various relatively rare disorders called "disconnection syndromes," since they involve loss of the connections or wires between major centers. For example, damage to the arcuate fasciculus, connecting Wernicke's area and the angular gyrus to Broca's area, can produce an aphasia in which the person can both comprehend and speak, since both Broca's area and Wernicke's area are intact, but cannot repeat what is said to him, since the auditory cortex and Wernicke's area are disconnected from the speech area, thus preventing the person from converting what he has heard into an identical spoken sentence.

The language system illustrates the high degree of specialization that our brains have achieved. Not only is this system located on only one side of the brain, but its components are relatively small areas of cortical tissue, each of which is dedicated to performing a particular type of language function. For the system as a whole to work properly, both the specialized cortical centers and the wiring that connects them must remain intact.

This system is frequently damaged in people who have suffered from stroke. As they recover, however, they may regain some language function even though part of the center may be destroyed or substantial amounts of wiring may be lost. Sometimes the remaining parts of the center learn to carry the whole burden. In addition, sometimes the brain figures out new wiring patterns, particularly for those components of the system that do have bilateral representation: the auditory cortex and the visual cortex. If a message cannot get through to Broca's area because damage has occurred to the wiring on the left side, messages may be sent to Broca's area through a "long circuit" instead of the usual short circuit, and speech may still occur. This would involve sending a message across the corpus callosum at the back of the brain, forwarding it on around through the right hemisphere, and sending it back through the corpus callosum at the front of the brain to Broca's area.

In some patients suffering from mental illness, the language system appears to be "broken" in some way. Patients suffering from schizophrenia provide some of the most vivid examples of abnormal language. One schizophrenic patient, asked what he thought about the energy crisis, replied:

> They're destroying too many cattle and oil just to make soap. If we need soap when you can jump into a pool of water, and then when you go to buy your gasoline, my folks always thought they could get pop, but the best thing to get is motor oil, and money. May as well go there and trade in some pop caps and, uh, tires, and tractors to car garages, so they can pull cars away from wrecks, is what I believed in.

This confused language is not unlike that produced by patients who have damage to Wernicke's area.

THE MEMORY SYSTEM

The memory system is different from all the other functional brain systems that we have examined so far in one important respect: It is localized in many different parts of the brain and almost certainly is not lateralized to only one hemisphere; in fact, for many years some scientists believed that memory could not be localized at all. Karl Lashley, a psychologist at Harvard, devoted most of his career to searching for the "engram," the symbolic figure through which memory traces might be encoded. Lashley produced injuries, or lesions, in many different parts of the brain in animal experiments. All he was able to demonstrate was that the ability to remember could not be damaged by injury to a specific part of the brain. Lashley reached the conclusion that memory is diffusely distributed throughout the brain.

Although Lashley's conclusion was essentially incorrect—memory traces for specific information *are* specifically localized—it is now easy to see why he was misled. Memory traces tend to be recorded bilaterally and in several places at the same time. Although the computer may be a poor model for the brain in some respects, in this instance it seems as if the brain's designer knew the rule that every wise computer hobbyist or professional follows: Remember to make a backup file.

In 1953, however, a fresh perspective was introduced when Scoville and Milner described the famous case of H.M. H.M. suffered from severe grand mal epilepsy that could not be controlled with high doses of medication. In the hope of stopping these seizures, William Scoville, a neurosurgeon, removed the inside half of the temporal lobe on each side of H.M.'s brain, the part of the temporal lobe that contains the hippocampus. After he recovered from this surgery, H.M. was found to have a severe, incapacitating memory impairment of a type called "anterograde amnesia": He could remember everything he had already learned, but could not learn anything new.

The case of H.M. has taught us several important facts about memory. First of all, it has indicated that memory functions *are* to some extent localized within the brain. The type of memory loss that H.M. experienced was a specific inability to learn new material. He retained good memory of events that occurred prior to the surgery. He also had normal intelligence, with an IQ of 118 as measured by the Wechsler Adult Intelligence Scale. He could speak and comprehend normally, and even understand complicated jokes. On the other hand, he was unable to remember anything that happened after the surgery for longer than one minute. It made no difference whether the new information was presented to him in words, by visual sensations, or by other senses such as touch. Even such catastrophic events as the death of his father were apparently forgotten within seconds after learning about them. Thus he remained frozen at some moment in time prior to his surgery. Everything that he encountered thereafter was a completely new event that he would always experience as new no matter how many times he encountered it. He had totally lost the ability to learn.

Following H.M., other similar cases have been noted, and we have come to realize that specific parts of the brain are dedicated to the process of learning new material. In addition to the hippocampus (the part damaged in H.M.), the mammillary bodies, the septal region of the limbic system, and part of the thalamus have also emerged as structures involved in memory. When damage occurs on only one side, memory usually remains intact, but when bilateral lesions occur, the memory deficit is complete.

Neuroscientists have come to conceptualize memory as a two-stage process. One type of memory is short-term memory. We use short-term memory, for example, when we hear a phone number, remember it briefly, dial it, and forget it in the course of conversing with the person we have called. Sometimes we want to remember things for longer periods of time. When we do this, we are said to have "learned" them. Put another way, a short-term memory has been "consolidated" and converted to a long-term memory.

The hippocampus, mammillary bodies, anterior thalamus, and septal region are probably all centers involved in converting short-term memory to long-term memory and storing it. Techniques such as rehearsal or repetition aid in the conversion of short-term memories to long-term, but neuroscientists have not yet determined definitively how this process actually occurs in the brain. Most research suggests that short-term memory involves setting up brief reverberating circuits through the electrical transmission of nerves, while long-term memory probably involves a more permanent process represented by actual physical changes in the brain, through the creation of new connections between nerve cells or through the creation of "memory molecules" that contain a code for each idea.

Thus, the story of the nature of memory is still evolving. According to our current state of knowledge, the memory system appears to consist of a set of discrete consolidation or storage centers arranged symmetrically on both sides of the brain, such as the hippocampus and mammillary bodies. If only one of these "files" is damaged, the individual is still able to remember normally, but if the files on both sides are destroyed, then he loses his ability to learn new material. On the other hand, short-term memories of specific auditory, visual, or other sensory perceptions are localized specifically but are widely distributed throughout the brain.

THE FRONTAL SYSTEM

While we know a great deal about the motor, sensory, and language systems, and quite a lot about the memory system, the frontal system is still a poorly understood frontier area. As we have seen from drawings and illustrations earlier in this chapter, the frontal lobes are the largest and most impressive parts of the brain. It is only natural to assume that such a large area would perform some important function, and for many years it was assumed that the frontal lobes must be a "seat of intelligence." During recent years, this view of the frontal lobes has been modified considerably. The frontal system now appears to be an important coordinator of emotion, volition, judgment, and creativity. Like the limbic system, and perhaps the language system or the memory system, it is a part of the brain that may become broken in those people suffering from what is popularly (and in some sense correctly) called a "nervous breakdown."

We can begin to understand the frontal system by looking at another famous historical case, that of Phineas Gage, described by Harlow in 1868. Phineas Gage was a dynamite worker who survived an explosion that drove an iron bar through the front of his head. Prior to the injury, he was an intelligent and pleasant person. After the injury, he began to behave in an inappropriate and childlike way. He was impulsive, unable to follow through on tasks that he planned, and showed poor social judgment by being irreverent and profane in inappropriate settings. Harlow assumed that the balance between his intellectual faculties and animal passions had been disturbed.

Although the case of Phineas Gage suggested that the frontal lobes might provide important clues concerning the nature of mental illness, since Gage's symptoms primarily involved personality and social behavior, the frontal lobes remained the "seat of the intellect" until the 1930s. In 1932 Brickner reawakened interest in the frontal lobes by describing another case similar to Phineas Gage. This patient, however, had had his frontal lobes removed surgically by the famous American neurosurgeon Walter Dandy. Like Phineas Gage, he displayed remarkable changes in his personality, becoming transformed from a shy, introverted individual into someone who was outgoing, boastful, and sometimes socially inappropriate. Yet he continued to have essentially normal intellectual function: He had a good memory, could speak and write normally, and could play games such as checkers.

A few years later Jacobsen and Fulton described the effects of removing both frontal lobes in two chimpanzees named Becky and Lucy. Like Phineas Gage and Brickner's patient, Becky and Lucy seemed to become different animals after the surgery. Prior to surgery they had been trained to perform several learning tasks, such as solving mazes. After the surgery they were also presented with various learning tasks, but they no longer became frustrated or upset when they were unable to solve them; instead, they seemed careless and happy.

Taken together, these various bits of research combined to suggest that the frontal lobes were more important as a "seat of emotions" than of intellectual abilities. D. O. Hebb confirmed this more strongly a few years later by reporting on four cases who had had large amounts of frontal tissue removed as a treatment for epilepsy. Since standardized IQ testing had become available, he administered these tests to patients before and after surgery, making the astonishing discovery that their IQs were not reduced even though large portions of the frontal lobes had been removed. Since IQ tests are designed to evaluate higher intellectual functions, it became clear that these could not be the primary activities of the frontal lobes. No doubt the work of Hebb is partly behind the erroneous commonplace that "large parts of our brains are essentially unused."

The Portuguese psychiatrist and neurologist Egas Moniz further advanced our understanding of the frontal lobes in 1936 by developing techniques of psychosurgery. Moniz was familiar with Brickner's report and the descriptions of Becky and Lucy. He speculated that cutting prefrontal fiber tracts in human beings might be useful in relieving the agitation of psychotic patients, particularly schizophrenics. Early reports by Moniz and others were highly favorable, and Moniz received a Nobel Prize in 1949 for developing the technique of prefrontal leucotomy (popularly known as lobotomy). Unfortunately, in the 1950s this technique was used overenthusiastically and overaggressively, especially in some state hospitals in the United States. It was later recognized that many patients, although relieved of severe agitation, also suffered from severe personality deficits not unlike those of Phineas Gage. Nevertheless, as Hebb had observed, their intelligence as measured by IQ testing was usually not decreased.

A more refined charting of the functions of the frontal system is currently under way, and the results indicate that the frontal system may be quite important in major mental illnesses such as schizophrenia or affective disorders. The frontal lobes contain the cingulate gyrus, which is part of the limbic system, and they also receive input from the hypothalamus and the basal ganglia, either directly or through the mediation of the thalamus. In turn, the frontal lobes also send messages back to these structures. Different parts of the frontal system are probably specialized to perform particular types of volitional and emotional functions. For example, damage to the bottom part of the frontal lobe, called the "orbital region" because it rests on the optic tracts, leads to a reduction in spontaneous behavior, to inappropriate sexual behavior such as masturbating in public, and to impaired social behavior and social judgment. Damage to the part of the frontal lobe right behind the forehead tends to make people inflexible and uncreative; they tend to get stuck in a particular way of solving a problem and to repeat their mistakes over and over. Damage to the outer convexities of the frontal lobes tends to affect motor and spatial abilities.

As we shall see in later chapters, research conducted in the past two to three years suggests that there are signs of damage to the frontal lobes in schizophrenia. These hints that the frontal system may be damaged in some schizophrenic patients are quite consistent with the symptoms noted in schizophrenia. As we observed in chapter 4, patients suffering from schizophrenia often display bizarre, socially inappropriate behavior and act unpredictably or impulsively. They also tend to have difficulty initiating spontaneous behavior, whether it be spontaneous speech or social interaction; and not unlike patients with frontal lesions, they may have poor grooming or hygiene. Much further research will be required to determine whether some schizophrenic patients do indeed have "broken" frontal systems or whether there is a breakdown in the communication between the frontal system and other important systems, such as the limbic system. The story of biological psychiatry during the next ten years will be the unraveling of the answers to these questions.

THE NEUROENDOCRINE SYSTEM

The command center of the neuroendocrine system resides in the hypothalamus, a tiny structure smaller than your fingertip that rests just below the thalamus and communicates with the pituitary gland. While nuclei in the brainstem control muscular activities such as breathing or heart rate, the hypothalamus serves as a mediator between the brain and body by regulating the endocrine system.

The endocrine system is a group of glands scattered throughout the body. It includes the thyroid, the adrenals, the part of the pancreas that produces insulin, and the sexual glands (testes in men and ovaries in women). The hypothalamus communicates with these various glands through substances called "hormones," which are chemical messengers that must travel through the bloodstream in order to reach the glands that they control. The hypothalamus receives continuous feedback from the organs of the endocrine system, which also produce hormones, and it uses this feedback to monitor the pituitary.

For example, one of the functions of the thyroid gland is to regulate body temperature. If the hypothalamus receives a message from sensors in the skin that the body feels cold, it will send out a substance called "thyrotropin-releasing factor" (TRF). This TRF goes to the pituitary, telling it to release TSH, thyroid-stimulating hormone (also called "thyrotropin"). The TSH then travels by the bloodstream to the thyroid, where it triggers the release of thyroid hormone into the blood, thereby giving the body a command to warm up.

Similar feedback loops are used to regulate the production of estrogen from the ovaries, androgen from the testes, and corticosteroids from the adrenal glands. In addition to all these functions, the hypothalamus also contains centers that regulate aggression, appetite, thirst, water balance, and growth rate, usually with the pituitary serving as an intermediary.

As we shall see in chapter 7, research during the past five to ten years has suggested that patients with affective disorder, particularly some types of depression, may be suffering from an imbalance in the hypothalamic-pituitary-adrenal axis. Many of the symptoms of affective disorder are consistent with these types of neuroendocrine abnormality, since they involve changes in appetite, sleep regulation, and adaptability to stress and change.

HEMISPHERIC SPECIALIZATION AND ASYMMETRY

As the previous review of functional systems in the brain indicated, many are crossed and lateralized. Most language functions occur only in the left hemisphere. The left hemisphere receives sensory information from receptors on the right side of the body and sends out commands for movement to the right side of the body; the right hemisphere interprets information from and sends motor commands to the left side. While the parietal region in the left hemisphere is chiefly concerned with integrating language functions, the parietal region in the right hemisphere specializes in visual-spatial information, such as the recognition of faces.

These facts have led some neuroscientists to speculate that the two hemispheres may also differ in overall "cognitive style." According to this theory, the left hemisphere is prone to specialize in verbal, analytic, and sequential processing, while the right hemisphere specializes in nonverbal, visual-spatial, intuitive, and gestaltlike processing. Individuals may differ from one another in cognitive style depending on which of their hemispheres tends to dominate. Sometimes people may use one hemisphere to solve certain kinds of problems and the other hemisphere to solve other kinds of problems. For example, the left-hemisphere approach to figuring out a missing word in a crossword puzzle would involve a systematic memory search for all words that would meet the required parameters, such as the number of letters and definition. A right-hemisphere approach to finding the missing word would be to sit in a relaxed manner until the answer suddenly appears.

Because schizophrenia frequently involves disorders of language and logical thought, some psychiatrists speculate that it is due to disease localized in the left hemisphere. On the other hand, since the affective disorders are primarily diseases of emotion, psychiatrists sometimes hypothesize that they are due to abnormalities of right-hemisphere structures or function. While interesting and theoretically appealing, these hypotheses are still largely unproved and probably are too simplistic.

In very recent years, however, interest in hemispheric specialization and asymmetry has been enhanced by the work of leading neuroscientists such as Norman Geschwind and Roger Sperry. Geschwind aroused great interest in hemispheric specialization when he demonstrated in 1968 that the human brain had an obvious structural asymmetry that had gone unnoticed for centuries. When the cerebral hemispheres are removed from the top of the temporal lobes, an area called the "planum temporale" (temporal plane) appears. In most human beings, this temporal plane is about three times larger on the left side than it is on the right. Since the left temporal region is heavily dedicated to language comprehension and production, one can infer that this structural enlargement reflects the left hemisphere's specialization in language.

If each of the hemispheres is specialized to perform particular and different kinds of functions, then when all works well they might frequently "talk" back and forth to one another and share their different special abilities, much like two scientific collaborators or two good friends. On the other hand, one might predict dire consequences if the two hemispheres are prevented from communicating with one another.

Again, the treatment of epilepsy has shed some light on this problem. Roger Sperry has studied a number of people who have been treated for intractable epilepsy through cutting the corpus callosum, that thick band of white-matter tracts that provides the connection between the two hemispheres, a procedure known as "commissurotomy" (cutting of the commissure). Surprisingly, these people showed little or no abnormality in cognitive function when evaluated routinely. When somewhat more subtle testing was done, however, clear abnormalities did emerge.

For example, the sense of smell is one of the few sensory modalities that is not crossed. When commissurotomized patients were presented with an odor in the right nostril, they were unable to name the odor, since information about the smell could not be communicated to the language system in the left hemisphere. They were able to point with the left hand to a picture of the object that they smelled, such as a peppermint stick, since the right hemisphere, which received the odor, was also able to control the left hand. But they could not point to the object with the right hand, since the left hemisphere was disconnected from information about the odor, and it is the left hemisphere that controls movement on the right side of the body.

A small body of research suggests that some patients with schizophrenia may have thickening of the corpus callosum, suggestive of an increase in the number of communicating fibers between the two hemispheres. Patients with this anatomic abnormality might be suffering from a "hyperconnection syndrome," causing their two hemispheres to be bombarded with more information than they are able to handle. This might lead to delusions arising from overinterpretation of sensory information or to hallucinations. This is another tantalizing theory that awaits investigation during the next few years. As chapter 7 describes in more detail, exciting new ways of visualizing the brain in living human beings have been developed during the past ten years and will be steadily refined during the next ten years. These techniques will help us determine whether there are in fact structural and functional brain abnormalities in schizophrenia and the affective disorders.

Organization of the Brain at the Cellular Level

So far we have looked at the brain to see what we can learn by examining it with the naked eye. We have examined various parts of its large-scale structure and learned how the functions of its various parts have been mapped through observing people who have had injuries to these areas, either through surgery or disease or both. This has been the world of the brain as seen by the anatomist and the clinician.

But one must also understand the brain at another level and from another perspective, moving from macrocosm to microcosm. One must learn to know the brain as it is seen with the aid of the microscope and the laboratory experiments of neuroscientists.

In this small-scale world of the brain, the building blocks are nerve cells. These nerve cells are of two types: neurons and glial cells. At the moment, most neuroscientists think the neurons do most of the work of the brain by formulating and transmitting all the messages that it carries. The glial (glue) cells are thought to be cementing, supporting, and nourishing structures for the neurons. In a few years, of course, some other function may be discovered for the glial cells, just as we have learned during recent years that the corpus callosum serves a much more important function than to hold up the two hemispheres.

CELL ARCHITECTURE

So many nerve cells are packed into the brain that we have no simple way to describe it in words. The brain has been estimated to contain 10,000,000,000,000 cells. Of these, 90 percent are glia. The remaining 10 percent, the neurons, form the communication centers and their wiring, and it is these cells in particular that we must learn to understand well.

Neurons differ in shape and appearance, depending on their purpose. Some are specialized to receive messages—the afferent (running in) neurons or bipolar neurons. Others are specialized to send out messages—the efferent (running out) neurons. Nevertheless, all neurons conform to a similar basic design, which is portrayed schematically in figure 11. The main work center of the neuron is the cell body, which contains the nucleus of the cell. The cell body is darker in appearance than the remainder of the cell, and when large numbers of cell bodies are packed together in the brain, a dark region appears —the now familiar cortical bark or major subcortical gray-matter command centers such as the basal ganglia. The cell bodies send out tiny fingers of branching fibers called "dendrites" (treelike structures). This treelike web around the cell body enormously increases its ability to receive information, since other cells can communicate either to the cell body itself or to its dendrites.

In addition to the dendrites, the cell body sends out a long, tubular projection that it uses to communicate with other neurons. This projection—the axon (axis)—is usually enclosed in a fatty sheath containing a substance called myelin that wraps around the axon and acts as an insulator. The axons are the "wires" of the nervous system. Some axons are relatively short, but there are axons whose cell bodies begin in the spinal cord and travel down to muscles in the foot—a length as long as one meter. The myelin sheath gives them a lighter appearance, and thus the axons constitute the white matter of the brain. This sheath is composed of glial cells called "Schwann cells" that wrap

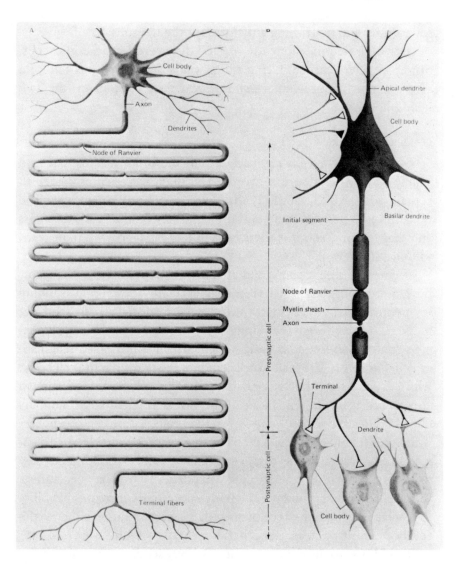

Fig. 11. **Structure of neurons.**

themselves around the neuron. The space between Schwann cells is called the "node of Ranvier." This organization permits electrical impulses to travel from the cell body to the end of the nerve by skipping from node to node, thus speeding up the rate at which messages travel. The end of the axon branches out into as many as 1,000 terminals. These terminals may end either on the cell bodies or dendrites of other neurons or on muscles of the face, arms, and legs.

Figure 11 shows the general structure of a neuron specialized for sending messages. If this neuron were specialized for receiving messages, it would have a somewhat different structure. The afferent, or receptor, neurons have axons that begin on sensory receptors such as those located in the eye, ear, or skin. They send messages to a cell body through an axon, which then sends out another long axon with branching terminals. Because these cells have two long axons, they are referred to as "bipolar neurons." In addition to afferent and efferent neurons, there are also many neurons whose main function is to provide connections between afferents and efferents. These types of cells are called "interneurons."

Different parts of the cortex contain different kinds of neurons arranged in somewhat different patterns. Information about the appearance and organization of nerve cells provided the earliest breakthroughs in the neurosciences. These discoveries were being made while Freud and Kraepelin were beginning their careers and then developing their own particular contributions to our understanding of the brain and mind, and were made possible through the development of special staining techniques that permitted brain cells to be seen clearly under the microscope. It was soon discovered that different kinds of stains would permit the eye to see different aspects of the neuron. This is shown in figure 12, which also indicates that the cortex may contain as many as eight different layers of cells. The Golgi stain darkens a few cell bodies but shows all their axons and dendrites. The Nissl stain shows cell bodies clearly but does not reveal any axons. The Weigert stain covers the myelin sheath and shows where axons are located.

Brodmann, a member of Kraepelin's department, used all these various staining techniques to develop what are called "cytoarchitectonic maps" of the cortex, demonstrating that different parts of the cortex had different patterns of cells with different layers more prominent in some areas than in others. Schematically, the cortex has six layers, with the outer four organized principally to receive messages and the inner two to send out messages. In some parts of the brain, however, such as the limbic system, the organization is clearly different: The limbic system contains only three layers and therefore seems structurally more primitive, leading it to be called the "paleocortex" (old cortex). Brodmann mapped over fifty distinct regions of the

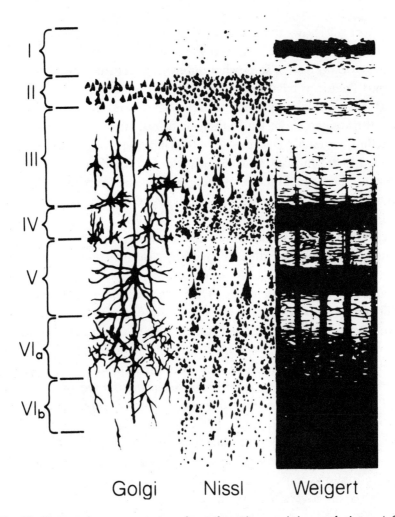

Fig. 12. Neuronal structures seen through various staining techniques (after Brodmann).

cortex on the basis of cell architecture. He did this work so carefully and precisely that modern behavioral neurologists continue to employ Brodmann's maps in order to understand the functional specialization of the brain.

Examples of Brodmann's maps appear in figure 13. On these maps we can find some areas familiar from the previous section. Area 4 is the motor strip, while area 3, 1, 2 is the somatosensory region. Areas 17, 18, and 19 constitute the visual cortex, while areas 41 and 42 are the primary auditory cortex. Within the language system, areas 44 and

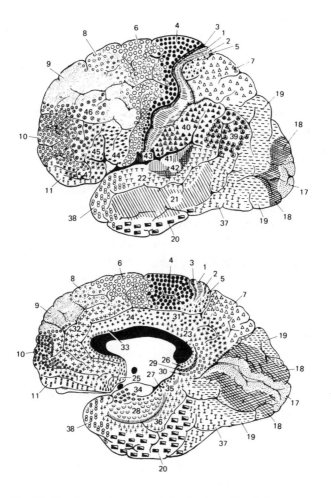

Fig. 13. **Brodmann's maps of the brain cells of the cortex.**

45 are Broca's area. Although Brodmann never won a Nobel Prize for his work (Golgi did), the continuing usefulness of his maps of cell architecture pays tribute to the importance of careful and detailed fact-collecting in the history of science.

COMMUNICATION BETWEEN NEURONS

By now the reader has probably developed a reasonably good visual and mental model of what the brain is really like: large numbers of specialized control centers composed of nerve-cell bodies connected to one another by wires (the axons) forming a complicated set of electrical circuits, all neatly packed within the skull. How do the messages actually get sent through those wires?

The messages are sent down the axons through a process of electrical conduction. When an axon is at rest, it is filled with and surrounded by a fluid containing a high concentration of electrically charged substances called ions, such as sodium (Na+), potassium (K+), and chloride (Cl−). When a message arrives at the axon telling it to fire, an event called an "action potential" occurs. The permeability of the membrane forming the axon changes, and this causes positively charged sodium ions, which have been floating around outside the membrane, to flow in, thereby triggering a large positive charge inside the cell. The larger the axon, the faster the message can move. Since large axons would take up a great deal of space inside the brain and cut down on its efficiency, nature evolved the technique of the myelin sheath and the node of Ranvier. The myelin sheath insulates the axon and increases the speed of conduction by as much as 100 times. Moreover, the exposure of the bare axonal membrane at the node of Ranvier permits the electrical impulse to travel by large jumps from node to node (called "saltatory conduction"), thereby further increasing the speed of transmission. Some important diseases of the nervous system, such as multiple sclerosis, do their damage primarily by destroying the myelin sheath. The loss of this important insulator in patches of white matter throughout the brain leads to widespread damage to the brain's circuitry, causing such symptoms as visual impairment, poor coordination, and slurred speech.

When the electrical impulse flowing down the axon reaches its end, it spreads out in hundreds of nerve terminals that communicate with the dendrites and cell bodies of many other neurons. The communication point between neurons is referred to as the "synapse" (junction). Much of the work in neuroscience during the past decades has been devoted to illuminating how nerve cells carry messages down the axon and how they communicate at synapses. During the 1930s, neuroscientists were divided into two factions: The physiologists, led by Sir John Eccles, argued that communication across the synapse was electrical; while the pharmacologists argued that the communication must be chemical. Research conducted from the 1950s to the present has indicated that both were right, although most transmission tends to be neurochemical.

Figure 14 portrays a stylized representation of an axon terminal and synapse. The negative electrical current is passing down the axon by hopping from node to node, eventually bringing a positive charge to the nerve terminal. Clustered at the end of the nerve terminal are hundreds of tiny sacs (synaptic vesicles) containing chemical substances referred to as "neurotransmitters." When they receive a strong positive charge, they interpret this as a message to release. The "release" command also requires the influx of positively charged calcium ions, which provides a way of modulating synaptic transmission. When the packets of neurochemicals (or quanta) receive the release message, the sacs surrounding them burst and neurochemical transmitters flow out into the synaptic cleft. There they interact with receptors on adjacent neurons. These receptors are highly specialized and understand messages only from particular types of neurochemi-

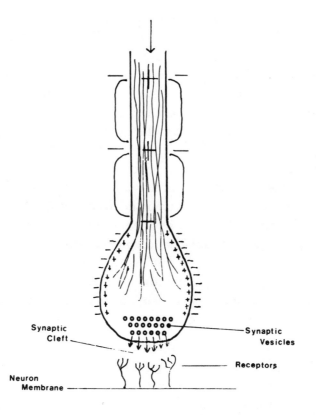

Fig. 14. Schematic representation of an axon and synapse.

cals. They can be thought of as a key and a lock—only a particular chemical can attach to a receptor to "unlock" it and give it a message.

As we shall see shortly, neurotransmitters of various types can carry different types of messages. Some are excitatory (that is, they encourage the development of action potentials), while others are inhibitory (they lower the cell's resting potential, thereby decreasing its ability to develop an action potential). While figure 14 portrays the synapse as if it were a simple one-to-one connection between neurons, in real life each neuron cell body or dendrite receives input from hundreds of nerve terminals. The receptor neuron will "decide" to fire only if it receives strong excitatory input from a number of different terminals.

The story of how the synapse works is a relatively recent one in the history of neuroscience, and it is still evolving. Once it was recognized that most neurotransmission was chemical, scientists began to explore which chemicals were being used to send messages. Only in the late 1960s and early 1970s were the laboratory techniques developed to map the locations of neurotransmitters in the brain. Earlier, Sir Henry Dale formulated a fundamental rule about synaptic transmission: Any given neuron uses the same transmitter substance at all of its synapses. During the past few years, exceptions to Dale's law have been discovered, but for the moment we will keep the story relatively simple. Following Dale's law, we can think of the brain as composed of cell groups that specialize in sending messages with different kinds of neurochemicals.

Much of the current research in neuroscience is devoted to identifying and charting the locations of neurotransmitters in the brain and learning how they interact with receptor sites in other neurons. Scientists have agreed to use a consistent set of rules in determining whether a particular chemical substance is actually a neurotransmitter. There are four criteria that a chemical substance must meet before it can be considered a neurotransmitter:

1. It is synthesized in the neuron.

2. It is present in the presynaptic terminal and is released in amounts sufficient to exert a particular effect on a receptor neuron.

3. When applied exogenously (as a drug) in reasonable concentrations, it mimics exactly the action of the endogenously released neurotransmitter.

4. A specific mechanism exists for removing it from its site of action, the synaptic cleft.

Following these criteria, eight substances have been accepted as neurotransmitters. These are classified into three main groups, as shown in table 3.

Table 3.
NEUROTRANSMITTERS CURRENTLY IDENTIFIED IN THE BRAIN

Cholinergic	Biogenic Amines	Amino Acids
Acetylcholine	Dopamine	γ-Aminobutyric
	Norepinephrine	Acid (GABA)
	Serotonin	Glycine
	Histamine	Glutamate

Many neuroscientists believe that the "break" in the brain leading to mental illness is a breakdown in neurotransmitter systems. As we shall see in chapters 8 and 9, which describe the search for drug treatments and the search for neurochemical causes, there are many hints that mental illness is due to chemical imbalances in the brain and that treatment involves correcting these chemical imbalances. Consequently, it is important to have a sense of the nature and location of at least some of these major neurotransmitter systems.

Acetylcholine was the first substance recognized as a neurotransmitter within the central nervous system. It appears almost everywhere in the brain, but has particularly high concentration in the basal ganglia and motor cortex. We know that many drugs used to treat mental illness interact in some way with acetylcholine, primarily by inhibiting it, although these interactions are considered to be side effects of the drugs rather than a major mechanism of action. These effects on acetylcholine are called "anticholinergic side effects."

Dopamine is the neurotransmitter that is thought to be excessively elevated in some patients suffering from schizophrenia. Many of the drugs used to treat schizophrenia decrease dopamine transmission. The dopamine system is portrayed in schematic form in figure 15. As that figure shows, dopamine tracts are located in three regions: the substantia nigra, the midbrain, and the hypothalamus. Parkinson's disease is due to loss of dopaminergic cells in the substantia nigra and is treated by providing supplemental dopamine in the form of L-dopa. The dopamine-containing cells of the midbrain project to the limbic

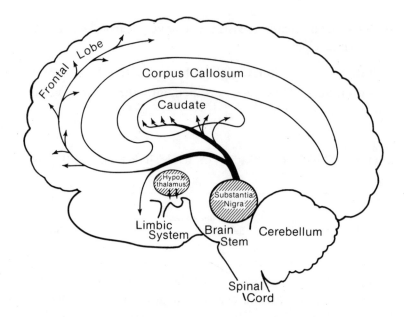

Fig. 15. **The dopamine system.**

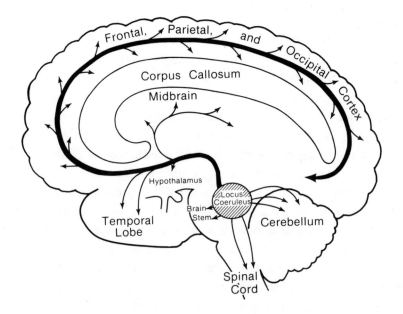

Fig. 16. **The norepinephrine system.**

cortex, thought to be the part of the brain disturbed in schizophrenia. The dopamine cells of the hypothalamus project to the pituitary, another important system in regulating emotional functions, such as response to stress and sexuality.

The neurotransmitter system that carries norepinephrine (also known as noradrenaline) is portrayed in figure 16. This system, also called the "noradrenergic system," begins in a small area of the brainstem and projects from there in a broad, netlike manner up through the midbrain and all over the cerebral cortex. It looks as if it must have some major modulating effect. This system is also important to the study of mental illness, since there are many hints from pharmacological and neurochemical research that patients suffering from depression may suffer from a deficit of norepinephrine.

Finally, the serotonin (or serotonergic) system is portrayed in figure 17. Like the norepinephrine system, the serotonin system begins in the brainstem and projects widely throughout the cerebral cortex, again looking as if it may have some diffuse regulatory function. It also has a heavy input to that well-used marriage chamber, the

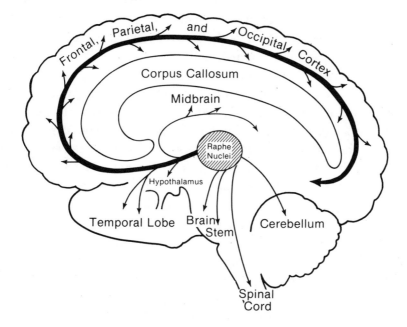

Fig. 17. The serotonin system.

thalamus. This system, too, is important in the study of mental illness. Some investigators have postulated that there are two subtypes of depression: one caused by abnormal norepinephrine balances and the other by abnormal serotonin balances. They postulate that although these depressions appear to be similar in their clinical symptoms, they are due to different chemical causes and likely to respond to different types of drugs.

The amino-acid transmitters are a group of substances that have a simpler chemical structure than those just described, and many of them are naturally occurring substances. For example, glutamate is an amino acid that many people put on food, especially Oriental food, in the form of monosodium glutamate, to enhance its flavor. This substance is particularly puzzling since there is fairly strong evidence that it is a neurotransmitter in the cerebellum and spinal cord, yet there is also evidence suggesting that it may have a toxic or destructive effect on neurons, particularly in children. As a consequence, the use of monosodium glutamate to flavor baby foods has been eliminated. Gamma-aminobutyric acid (GABA) is synthesized from glutamate. It almost certainly functions in some areas as an inhibitory neurotransmitter.

In very recent years, a variety of neuroactive peptides (chains of amino acids) have also been identified. Some of these are regulatory hormones released by the hypothalamus to govern the actions of the pituitary, such as thyrotropin-releasing hormone (TRH). Another family of neuroactive peptides that has commanded great attention recently is the endorphins and the enkephalins. These peptides, which do not meet all the criteria for neurotransmitters, tend to perform opiatelike actions in the brain. They attach to groups of receptors scattered throughout the central nervous system that are referred to as "opiate receptors" and appear to have an important function in modulating the perception of pain. These opiate receptors are located in areas thought to be important to the development of mental illness —the thalamus, the amygdala, and the caudate, to mention only a few.

They are important theoretically because they suggest that the central nervous system contains its own endogenous opioids as well as receptors specialized to receive messages from a class of drugs that are often used to treat pain and which produce euphoria as a side effect: opiates such as morphine or heroin. They have increased our awareness of how specific the receptor regions in the brain may be, and have led us to wonder how many other receptors exist that may be prepared to accept messages from chemicals not known to occur naturally in our bodies. Finally, because the opiate receptors are located in the limbic system and basal ganglia, a few investigators have used substances such as the endorphins to treat schizophrenia, introducing the possibility that yet another mechanism besides excessive dopamine may account for the occurrence of schizophrenia.

One cannot leave the subject of neurotransmitters without some further discussion of that other side of the synapse: the receptor. Receptors were presumed to exist long before they were actually discovered. Research in recent years has indicated that the "receptor" is a specific site on the neuronal membrane that contains a particular type of protein. This protein is specifically constructed to receive messages from particular kinds of neurotransmitters. As this is studied further, the receptor is turning out to be a very complicated piece of small machinery. It appears to have a variety of components that perform different functions: One part of it binds neurotransmitters; another may change membrane permeability; yet another may communicate with the inside of the cell membrane to send a message; and yet another may act as a modulator.

We now know that some drugs may increase or decrease the sensitivity of particular receptors, and this may either cause side effects or explain their mechanism of action. For example, prolonged use of neuroleptics, drugs used to treat schizophrenia, may eventually lead to receptors that are oversensitive, thereby producing an important unwanted side effect: tardive dyskinesia (a movement disorder to be discussed in chapter 8). On the other hand, other psychoactive drugs, like Valium, may bind to the modulating component in the GABA receptor, preventing it from doing its work and giving GABA free rein as an inhibitor. This mechanism would explain why a drug like Valium acts as a tranquilizer.

THE REVOLUTION IN NEUROSCIENCE

The thoughtful reader may long ago have said to himself: This is not the story of a revolution; this is the story of the slow, steady building of fact upon fact and truth upon truth over the past one hundred years. That, of course, is true. *Revolution* is perhaps much too colorful and extreme a word to describe this slow, steady growth in knowledge.

Nonetheless, investigators currently working in the neurosciences, particularly those interested in the relationship between neuroscience and mental illness, do regard the work of the past ten to twenty years as revolutionary in their impact. It is a revolution not so much in terms of what we know as in how we perceive what we know. This shift in perception suggests that we need not look to theoretical constructs of the "mind" or to influences from the external environment in order to understand how people feel, why they behave as they do, or what becomes disturbed when people develop mental illness. Instead, we can look directly to the brain and try to understand both normal behavior and mental illness in terms of how the brain works and how the brain breaks down. The new mode of perception has created the exciting feeling that we can understand the causes of mental illness in terms of basic biological mechanisms. If we can understand how those mechanisms have "broken," we will understand the cause and perhaps develop better forms of treatment.

Those discoveries concerning the causes and treatments of mental illness are occurring now and will continue to occur during the next ten to twenty years. The problem will probably not be solved by a single person or a single hypothesis, as was the riddle of DNA through the discovery of the double helix. Instead, it will be a collaborative effort involving contributions of scientists from many different fields, including neurochemistry, neuropharmacology, neuroanatomy, neuropathology, behavioral neurology, and psychiatry. Perhaps this slow, steady growth of knowledge through the collaboration of various disciplines should more precisely be called the "evolution" in neuroscience. Nevertheless, the *spirit* of a revolution —the sense that we are going to change things dramatically, even if the process requires a number of years—is very much present.

6

THE REVOLUTION IN DIAGNOSIS:

The Search for New Kinds of Illness

Great changes there must be, for a revolution cannot accomplish itself
without great changes; yet order there must be, for without order a
revolution cannot accomplish itself by due course of law.

—MATTHEW ARNOLD,
Culture and Anarchy

The process of learning to be a doctor involves learning how to do
two things: to make a diagnosis and to give treatment for the illness
diagnosed. The greater of the two is learning how to diagnose. But
giving treatment often seems more dramatic.

While most doctors do both diagnosis and treatment, different
specialties may stress one or the other. The surgeon, for example, is
an expert in treatment. We tend to think of him as a man in his late
thirties, attired in greens, usually handsome, certainly outspoken and
aggressive. He is decisive, perhaps abrasive, and often abrupt. Patients fear and admire him. He is a doer. He is glamorous. Even an
ordinary operation—removing a gallbladder or an appendix—has an
aura of mystery about it. The surgeon works on a patient who is
asleep, unconscious, who has literally put herself *in his hands.* He cuts
open her body, makes her bleed and stops the blood almost simultaneously, examines her internal organs, identifies the source of disease,
cuts it out, and sews her back together again. Small wonder that his
work seems miraculous. It *is.* And the development of new surgical
techniques, such as open-heart surgery and transplantation of organs,
seems like divine creation. To remove a healthy kidney from a donor
and use it to replace the diseased kidney of another person is to

perform a priestlike or godlike function. The donor has made a voluntary sacrifice of a part of her body, taken a risk, and submitted to pain in order to give to another. The recipient may be freed from bondage to a machine and given a new life. The surgeon who performs the rite of transplantation, using his technical ability to remove organs, to keep them alive outside a human body, and then to place them in another human body, must have almost superhuman confidence and skill.

By comparison, the work of the diagnostician seems relatively drab and dull. But it is not. In fact, it is the exploratory adventure of medicine. Without the diagnostician, the surgeon could not survive, as he is usually the first to admit. The diagnostician is the pathfinder, the detective, the solver of riddles, the spy. His task is to discover what is wrong with the patient so that the proper treatment can be administered. Before the man in greens can wield his scalpel, a person in a white coat with a stethoscope, a microscope, or an X-ray must precede him. (The stereotype of this person is the kindly white-haired man with a sympathetic smile and a fatherly hand on the patient's shoulder. But, recognizing that medicine has become more egalitarian, let's make him a kindly woman instead.)

If the surgeon is spectacular, the diagnostician is ingenious. She too learns to look inside people, but in ways that are imaginative and noninvasive. She listens to heart sounds, palpates blood vessels, studies the color of the skin and the texture of the hair, and pushes on the abdomen searching for abnormal masses. She learns what is inside the body by looking at small samples of its contents under a microscope —learning by inference from blood or urine or spinal fluid what the surgeon sees directly. She asks questions in order to determine what symptoms the patient has had and whether they have changed by getting better or worse. She uses a wide range of X-ray procedures that permit her to see inside people's heads, hearts, and stomachs, simply by taking pictures that are sometimes enhanced by having them swallow special fluids or by injecting various "dyes" into their veins or arteries.

Everyone admires a surgeon. The diagnostician is a doctor's doctor. In medical school, students quickly notice that the word *diagnosis* is said in somewhat reverential tones. To most people, *diagnosis* is just a technical term that doctors use, but to a doctor this word describes his most serious, exciting, and even sacred task. It means literally "to know about, to know through, to understand" (Greek *dia* = about, through, across; *gnosis* = know). The apprentice doctor soon learns to admire and respect the skills of the more experienced diagnosticians who train him. They teach him how to collect thousands of tiny pieces of information, sift through them, pick out the important facts, and put them together to tell an accurate story of the patient's illness. To watch a great diagnostician interview, examine, and describe what she sees is as thrilling as watching the technical skills of a great surgeon. The excitement of diagnosis is the excitement of the detective story. While the surgeon is a doer, the diagnostician is a thinker, a seer, a prophet. She studies the past and predicts the future. She sees with her mind rather than her eyes. That, too, is a miracle.

The psychiatrist is first and foremost a diagnostician, one who explores the greatest uncharted territory remaining in medicine: the dark continent of the disordered brain. Her work is a journey into the heart of darkness. It is a darkness of uncertainty, for we are still discovering how to recognize and define the specific diseases that afflict the human brain. It is a darkness of suffering, because mental illness causes some of the worst anguish that human beings can experience. The psychiatrist has a bittersweet task. She works in perhaps the most exciting field in medicine; each day may be a voyage of discovery, an opportunity to observe some new fact or identify some new disease. But if she blends humane sympathy with scientific curiosity, she suffers vicariously along with her patients as she puts herself in their places and tries to understand what they think and feel. Her task requires courage and imagination in addition to curiosity and wisdom.

Psychiatric Diagnosis Before Kraepelin

Like other illnesses, the major mental illnesses have probably been present from the time that the brain of *Homo sapiens* assumed something resembling its present form. The earliest recorded references are in the medical texts of Pharaonic Egypt, written in hieroglyphics on papyrus as early as 1900 B.C. These texts indicate that Egyptian physicians observed and recognized many symptoms of mental illness, and almost invariably assumed that they were due to physical causes, most frequently to some kind of abnormality in the heart:

> As to the driving of the mind, it is that probably the blood coagulates in the heart.
> As the mind is kneeling (breaking down): this means that this mind is constricted and his heart becomes small. It is that the heart is hot and weary at each level and is fastidious.
> As to his mind is dark and he tastes his heart: this means that his mind is contracted, there being darkness in his belly, and he makes the deed to conserve his mind.

These descriptions from the Eber papyrus indicate that the Pharaonic Egyptians recognized symptoms of illnesses such as depression or schizophrenia. The descriptions are incomplete and the treatments are hardly modern, but psychiatric symptoms are accorded the same importance as other medical symptoms. One cannot help but be impressed by the concern about the existence of mental illnesses recorded 40 centuries ago. Monumental art, scenes of love and ambition, and incontrovertible evidence of the universality of death and disease reside together among the oldest remnants of civilized humanity.

The earliest extensive descriptions of mental illnesses derive from classical times. Two different kinds of sources give us parallel perspectives. On the one hand, there are didactic medical texts that tell us how Greek and Roman physicians perceived mental illness. On the other hand, we also have the literary portrayals of classical tragedy and comedy.

The medical texts indicate quite clearly that classical physicians approached mental illness as a type of physical disease. In fact, descriptions of mental illnesses are intertwined with descriptions of other illnesses as if no great differentiation were made between mind and body. Mania and melancholy are discussed in the midst of pneumonia and apoplexy. Hippocrates, the "Father of Medicine," who wrote the Hippocratic Oath that physicians take upon graduation from medical school as part of their rite of initiation into the responsibilities of caring for others, definitely believed that the brain was the source of thoughts and emotions and that most mental illness was due to malfunction of the brain. In discussing epilepsy, which some before him saw as a "sacred disease" that might reflect divine possession, Hippo-crates states: "It seems to me to be no more divine and no more sacred than other diseases, but, like other affections, it springs from natural causes. . . ."

The types of mental illness that the classical Greeks recognized are strikingly similar to those still recognized today. In fact, much of our modern terminology derives from the classical Greeks. Mental ill-nesses that they described include mania, melancholia, hysteria, and phrenitis. Their mania corresponds roughly to modern schizophrenia and mania; their melancholia to modern depression; their hysteria to modern somatization disorder; and their phrenitis to the delirium that occurs during some infections and fevers. While their classifications and terms are strikingly similar, their explanations about causes and treatments of mental illnesses seem rather quaint. Hysteria was some-times described as a disease occurring primarily in women and due to a wandering uterus that slipped loose from its moorings, drifting upward to cause subjective suffocation and other symptoms; it was treated by pleasant fumes in the area of the vagina to attract the uterus back toward its natural home.

In classical times diseases were often thought to result from imbal-ances in the four fluids (or humors) found in the body: blood, phlegm, yellow bile, and black bile. Mild changes in the balances among these four types of fluids (which corresponded to the four "elements" recognized at the time: air, water, fire, and earth) led people to have different personalities or temperaments; thus they might be sanguine, phlegmatic, choleric, or melancholic. Severe imbalances led to dis-eases—depression or melancholy, for example, was due to an excess of black bile. These imbalances could be corrected by removing the excessive fluid whenever possible. Since blood was the most accessible fluid, bloodletting tended to be the most common treatment.

While Galen, Hippocrates, Soranus of Ephesus, and other classical physicians were teaching their students how to recognize and treat diseases, the poets were portraying the same diseases in literary form. We cannot say, of course, whether the poets knew of the medical teachings of the time and were consciously portraying specific types of disease, or whether they were sketching from life with a few em-bellishments from imagination. In any case, classical tragedy testifies eloquently that the Greeks recognized and feared mental illnesses.

Euripides' Medea, for example, appears to suffer from a severe melancholia, partly precipitated by her husband Jason's desertion, that makes life seem meaningless, cruel, and worthless. In this state of bitter despair, her impaired judgment leads her to commit a terrible act of destruction: She murders her children. The *Bacchae* of Euripides portrays a similarly horrifying murder, spurred by a different kind of madness. Agave, mother of King Pentheus, is a worshiper of the god Dionysus and is in a manic ecstasy. When Pentheus goes into the hills to reprimand her and the other Bacchic revelers, her psychotic vision perceives him as a wild animal, rather than a human being. She attacks him, tears off his head, and does a manic dance of joy while she carries it above her on a spear.

Ordinary Greeks may have been less tragically violent when stricken with madness, but they no doubt had similar illnesses; the basic groupings of symptoms seen in these characters of Euripides are not unlike those encountered by modern psychiatrists. The fact of mental illness seems to remain more or less constant. Only our perception of it seems to change.

The classical period was a time of enlightenment with respect to mental illness. The Greeks saw the various forms of madness as forms of physical illness, involuntary and requiring humane medical treatment. After the classical era, however, there was a long period of relative cruelty and misunderstanding. During the Christian era, mental illness was seen at best as something to ignore or avoid and at worst as something to punish and destroy. No medical texts are extant from the early medieval period, but literary and historical evidence indicates that the absence of texts does not bespeak the absence of illness. Saint Augustine has confessed to his struggles with the hopelessness and despair of depression; Saint John of the Cross and other mystics have written of the dark night of the soul, a powerful metaphor for melancholy. There are also hints of manic elation: Saint Joan listened to her voices and led France and herself to military glory, and Saint Theresa described her ecstatic mystical visions. The fate of Saint Joan indicates, however, the risks to which any form of deviance was subject. Her voices, it was decided at Rouen, were heard by a terrible heretic, who was best punished by being terribly burned.

In fact, during the early Renaissance era, the most frequently cited "medical text" concerning mental illness is a book about witchcraft, not medicine: the *Malleus Maleficarum (Hammer of Witches)*, written by two Dominican monks. This text described in detail how to recognize and prove that a person was indeed involved in witchcraft and possessed by the devil. The *Malleus* is based on the belief that various delusions and hallucinations are products of a fevered imagination that bespeaks involvement with satanic forces; such involvement is anti-Christian and heretical and therefore should be punished. As cases of possession and witchcraft are described, it is clear that most represent various forms of mental illness. People suffering from psychotic depressions who are deluded that they have committed unpardonable crimes; schizophrenics who experience the torments of hallucinatory voices; men and women who experience various kinds of sexual difficulties and preoccupations—all are seen as cases of possession. The Medieval and early Renaissance obsession with the supernatural made it unthinkable that these might be illnesses due to natural or physical causes.

It is easy to recoil from this era in self-righteous horror and to summarily condemn the authors of the *Malleus* and their many followers. If one puts oneself in their position, however, it seems clear that the persecutors of the mentally ill probably experienced as much mental anguish as their victims, if not as much physical anguish. They lived in a time when evil forces were thought to lurk everywhere. A tiny error in judgment, an accidental encounter with a devil masquerading in human form, perhaps even an excessive desire to associate with the opposite sex might lead to loss of one's immortal soul. Perceptions of the world ranged from guarded suspicion to full-blown paranoia. An angry glance from a neighbor might infect one's dairy cow, or even oneself, with a fatal illness. The forgetful, toothless old woman seen yesterday at the market might be corrupting one's mind with sinful sexual desires. The only way to protect society was to quickly and efficiently destroy anyone who might harbor demonic forces. Like germs, chemicals, and radiation in our society, demonic forces were seen everywhere by the medieval mind.

This view did not disappear along with the Middle Ages, however. As late as the seventeenth century, James VI of Scotland, soon to become James I of England and Scotland, was writing a treatise on demonology that differed little from the *Malleus Maleficarum* except that it was written in the vernacular. As the Inquisition and the Wars

of Religion receded, so did the fires in which witches were burned—
but not the prisons in which they were housed, along with the poor
and the mentally retarded.

Until the late eighteenth century, the classical interest in classifying, describing, studying, and treating various forms of mental illness
was almost totally lost. The rest of medical science, however, was
advancing. Human anatomy was mapped, the circulation of the blood
described, and miraculous drugs (like digitalis) discovered. The scientific revolution was under way, and medicine enjoyed many benefits
from its empirical and progressive point of view. But this progress did
not extend to the serious mental illnesses, although scientific interest
in the neuroses began to develop. The insane were herded off to
prisons along with debtors and criminals and chained to their walls.
Medical treatment, whether humane or inhumane, was often not even
considered. It is no doubt from this long period, extending from
classical times through the eighteenth century, when the insane were
largely outside the province of medicine, that we have derived so
much ingrained prejudice and fear about mental illness. We have
nearly two millennia of ignorance to overcome, with only two centuries of relative enlightenment balanced against them.

The Modern Era of Psychiatry

Some glimmerings of light did exist during these dark ages of
psychiatry. During the era when the *Malleus Maleficarum* dominated
most people's thinking, voices did speak out in protest. For example,
the Englishman Reginald Scot wrote a book called *The Discovery of
Witchcraft* in the early seventeenth century to prove that "the impacts
and contracts of witches with devils and all infernal spirits or familiars
are but erroneous novelties and imaginary conceptions." The English
physician Timothy Bright wrote *A Treatise of Melancholy* in which he
described symptoms of affective disorder in great detail, including a
tendency for some people to cycle between mania and depression,
thus foreseeing the concept of bipolar affective disorder without realizing it. The Swiss physician Felix Platter devoted his life to visiting
the prisons where the mentally ill were housed and developing a
classification system to describe their various symptoms. Further, as
was the case during classical and medieval times, the great literature

of the Renaissance and seventeenth century provides detailed descriptions of various types of mental illness: Hamlet's bipolar affective disorder, Lear's progressive memory loss and dementia, Ophelia's psychotic depression and suicide, the melancholy of Donne and Burton, and the schizophreniclike ramblings of Poor Tom in *King Lear.*

Nevertheless, the modern era of psychiatry had its beginnings only in the late eighteenth century. Then, along with the American and French revolutions, there was also a revolution in the way people perceived the mentally ill. Under the leadership of physicians like Pinel in France, Tuke in America, Chiarugi in Italy, and Langermann in Germany, mental illnesses were no longer seen as stigmatizing and degrading. These men all marched into their respective Bedlams and freed the insane from their chains. Figure 18 shows a famous picture of Pinel freeing the insane in the Salpêtrière in Paris. It symbolizes the dawn of the modern era in psychiatry.

What the Renaissance of interest in classical learning did not do for the mentally ill, the Enlightenment did. The eighteenth-century Enlightenment introduced such principles as the dignity of the individual human being, tolerance for variety and deviance, a healthy

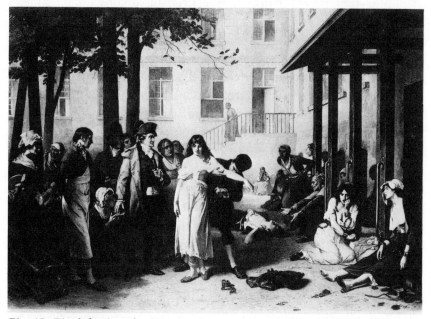

Fig. 18. Pinel freeing the insane. (Contempory photogravure of painting by Tony Robert-Fleury, 1876. *Clements C. Fry Collection. Yale Medical Library*)

skepticism about the supernatural, and a reverence for the empirical observation of nature. Not only was science valued, but people for the first time began to talk about "social science." The stage was set for the development of modern sociology, psychology, and psychiatry.

Medicine, the discipline from which psychiatry developed, was also in a period of growth. Scientists were investigating the relationship between the brain and the peripheral nerves ("the sinewy threads my brain lets fall," as John Donne much earlier had called them). However erroneously, Gall and his fellow phrenologists were attempting to map the locations of brain functions. Principles from other sciences, such as mechanics and electricity, were applied to medicine. The old theory of the humors was supplanted by a "solidist" orientation that emphasized that most diseases were due to abnormalities in particular organs. Instead of having "vapors" due to imbalances in their "humors," people began to have attacks of "nerves." Old terms like *mad* and *insane* were supplanted by new terms such as *neurosis* and *psychosis,* which reflected a more scientific understanding of the type of disease or disorganization that was occurring.

While some things changed, others remained constant. The mentally ill were unfortunately abundant in eighteenth- and nineteenth-century Europe and America, just as they had been in earlier times. In fact, they were more obvious both to society and to physicians once they had been freed from their chains. The situation was probably not unlike the results of the widespread discharge of the mentally ill from long-term-care hospitals in the United States during the 1960s and 1970s. Both physicians and the general populace were made painfully aware of the pervasive presence of mental illness in society.

Much of the effort of eighteenth- and nineteenth-century scientific psychiatry involved the careful description of the symptoms that patients displayed. It was hoped that in this way, improved methods for defining and classifying various types of mental illness could be discovered. A second goal was to understand the nature of the diseases in terms of the underlying bodily disturbances causing them. In other branches of medicine, clear, specific types of diseases with characteristic symptoms and outcomes were well recognized—apoplexy, consumption, pleurisy, and plague, for example. Doctors specializing in the care of the mentally ill, however, saw thousands of patients but had no clear consensus about how to diagnose their specific diseases. They were searching for a coherent diagnostic system, particularly one that made sense in terms of identifying the causes of the diseases and predicting outcome.

As noted earlier, the search for specific types of mental disease was finally fulfilled through the achievements of Emil Kraepelin. Drawing many ideas from his predecessors, Kraepelin developed the concepts of manic-depressive insanity and dementia praecox (schizophrenia). He did what many medical clinicians and teachers would love to do: He discovered new diseases (although, unlike Parkinson's disease, Alzheimer's disease, and Huntington's chorea, the disorders he discovered do not immortalize him through carrying his name). In addition to these two major illnesses, he described several others, such as psychoses occurring in late life ("paraphrenia") and disorders characterized primarily by delusional thinking with relative preservation of other functions ("paranoia"). His way of classifying mental diseases has remained in use since he invented it nearly 100 years ago.

Kraepelin's biological approach was admired and widely used in most of Europe and also planted some modest roots in American psychiatry. The ideas did have some fallow ground to fall on. American psychiatry has always had a modest tradition of studying and treating serious mental illnesses, with an effort to do so humanely. Benjamin Rush, one of the leaders of the American Revolution and a signer of the Declaration of Independence, was also a physician who was interested in serious mental illnesses. He was a leader both in establishing facilities to treat the mentally ill in the United States and in advocating a medical approach to mental illness. As America grew, state mental hospitals were created to care for the seriously ill. Some of these, called "psychopathic hospitals," were especially designed for the triple purposes of treatment, teaching, and research. The superintendents and doctors in many of the state hospitals and psychopathic hospitals maintained a medical orientation and fostered biological research.

As we saw in earlier chapters, however, the mainstream of American psychiatry became psychodynamic and psychoanalytic, abandoning the more biologically oriented Kraepelinian approach. In the 1950s, when manpower and money were invested in psychiatry for the first time on a large scale by the federal government, most of these resources went to psychiatry with a psychoanalytic orientation. Biological psychiatrists were not nonexistent during the 1950s and 1960s, but they were certainly not abundant. They were a disdained or disadvantaged minority. The intellectually curious person who decided to go into psychiatry usually did so because he wanted to become an analyst. He wanted to avoid the seriously ill, the state hospitals, the sight of blood, and an apparently outdated Germanic emphasis on the importance of diagnosis.

The Neo-Kraepelinian Revival

The psychoanalytic point of view tends to stress the importance of studying symptoms and complaints, but not the importance of studying diseases. The causes of symptoms are understood in terms of underlying psychodynamics, not in terms of biological disruption. An alternate point of view began to be stressed again in the 1950s and 1960s by a group of psychiatrists who sought to revive and reintroduce a more biological or medical orientation. Because they used Kraepelin rather than Freud as their rallying point, they are often referred to as the "Neo-Kraepelinians."

The Neo-Kraepelinian revival is usually said to have begun through the work of a small group of psychiatrists who taught at Washington University in St. Louis during the 1950s: Eli Robins, Samuel Guze, George Winokur, and the many students they trained. During the flowering of psychodynamic thinking, these psychiatrists saw themselves as an embattled minority trying to maintain the attachments of psychiatry to medical science and to neuroscience. They were working to introduce into American psychiatry a Germanic or British tradition that stressed the importance of diagnosis and the search for a biological cause of mental illness. During the 1950s and 1960s, the Neo-Kraepelinians were often ridiculed by "mainstream" American psychiatry for espousing a rigidly empirical or biological point of view and ignoring psychodynamic principles. During the 1970s, several factors converged to change this state of affairs. The time was ripe for the revolution that is occurring in the 1980s.

A crucial factor has been the development of new drug therapies. As chapter 8 describes in more detail, the care of the seriously ill has been dramatically affected by these new drugs, which have provided techniques for diminishing or even eliminating the symptoms of major illnesses such as schizophrenia or depression. These new drugs led to a resurgence of interest in the definition and diagnosis of major mental illnesses for several reasons. First of all, some of them appear to work for some specific illnesses and not for others. For example, the same drugs usually cannot be used to treat both schizophrenia and depression. Just as the internist must decide whether a patient has pneumococcal pneumonia or viral pneumonia because he will prescribe different drugs for these different illnesses, so too the psychiatrist found himself confronted with having to decide whether to use imipramine because the patient was suffering from depression or Thorazine because the patient had schizophrenia. If he made the wrong diagnosis, the patient would not get better and might even get worse. Second, the new drugs began to suggest hypotheses about the causes of mental illness and new methods for exploring their causes. The science of neurochemistry could be applied more easily to research in mental illness, since the drugs could be used in animal research to examine their effects on neurotransmitter systems. Third, the new drugs led many clinically oriented psychiatrists to become more interested in treating the seriously ill, because they at last had effective treatments to offer. The treatment of schizophrenia was no longer synonymous with chronic institutionalization in a state hospital.

Another crucial factor leading to a reemergence of interest in medical approaches to diagnosis and in biological psychiatry was the growth of the neurosciences. As chapter 4 has indicated, during the late nineteenth and early twentieth centuries, brain structure and function have gradually been systematically mapped in increasing detail. In particular, during recent years we have learned more about higher cortical functions, such as volition and memory, that are often impaired in serious mental illnesses. Neurochemistry, neuroendocrinology, and neuropharmacology have all provided additional clues concerning the causes of mental disorders. Suddenly, the curious young person interested in exploring new frontiers—the person who was likely to become a psychoanalyst during the 1950s—could see new vistas opening up in biological psychiatry. The tools for making discoveries about the relationship between the brain and mental illness were not available in the 1950s, but they are today. The person who wants to discover the causes of major mental illnesses such as schizophrenia must proceed from a medical model and assume that they are diseases. And he must be concerned with careful diagnosis, because he wants to discover the specific causes of specific diseases.

Still another factor that helped to extend the Neo-Kraepelinian revival during the 1970s and 1980s was frustration among the mass of practicing psychiatrists about the imprecision of their diagnostic approaches and their difficulties in communicating with one another. The psychodynamic approach tended to emphasize that the truth about what was wrong with the patient was not obvious and usually lay beneath the surface. Unfortunately, psychiatrists often could not agree about what they observed, since what lay beneath the surface was relatively subjective. At its best, this approach led to challenging intellectual debates. At its worst, it led to confusion and nonproductive controversy. Disagreements about diagnosis and management were too often settled by an appeal to tradition, seniority, or authority, rather than by an appeal to facts. In public situations involving expert opinions, such as legal cases, psychiatrists could always be found to take opposing views, much to the embarrassment of the field as a whole. Even in private communication, such as referrals between doctors in different cities, clinicians were never sure that one person's diagnosis of schizophrenia was the same as another's. Consequently, psychiatrists felt a great need for a better approach to diagnosis, one that would be more objective, precise, and reliable.

American concern about improving the precision of diagnosis was greatly enhanced during the 1970s by the results of two large cross-national studies of psychiatric diagnosis. These were the International Pilot Study of Schizophrenia (IPSS) and the US-UK Study. The IPSS was designed to study the symptoms of schizophrenia in various parts of the world. Under the leadership of several innovative British psychiatrists, standard methods of evaluating and interviewing patients were developed and applied to patients in many different countries, such as the United States, Great Britain, Taiwan, Colombia, and the USSR. As the research progressed, it became apparent that two countries stood out as somewhat unusual in their diagnostic practice: the U.S. and the USSR. Both tended to have broader concepts of schizophrenia than any of the other countries involved in the study. Discovering themselves to have rather strange bedfellows, Americans began to examine their diagnostic practices more critically.

The US-UK Study added to the concern. In this study, British and American psychiatrists looked at videotaped interviews of the same patients. Again, it was noted that American psychiatrists tended to disagree with the diagnoses of British psychiatrists and in particular to diagnose schizophrenia more frequently. Americans began to wonder if their diagnostic practices might not be out of step with the rest of the world. They began to look for ways to improve diagnostic agreement between clinicians, technically known as "reliability of diagnosis."

Part of the solution to the problem was contributed by the Neo-Kraepelinians of Washington University. In an effort to improve the precision of diagnoses used in their research on the genetics of mental illness, they developed a standardized set of definitions for the common mental illnesses. Unlike the definitions that appeared in textbooks or the descriptions that you read in chapter 4, these standardized definitions specified exactly which symptoms must be present and how many were required in order to make a particular diagnosis. In other words, they established *criteria* for making various diagnoses.

Although this approach might seem simple and obvious, it was a relatively new and creative idea. Reliability of diagnosis, while a particularly great problem in psychiatry, has also been a problem in the field of medicine in general. Whenever an illness is conceptually complicated, clinicians have difficulty agreeing about its presence. Which symptoms and how many must a patient have for her doctor to be certain that she has multiple sclerosis, whiplash, or migraine headache? If diagnosis can be confirmed through a simple laboratory test, as in the case of most infectious diseases, then the diagnostic process is simpler and more reliable. When no such tests are available, boundaries tend to become blurred and unclear. But the specification of precise criteria for making these difficult diagnoses ensures that clinicians will agree with one another reasonably well. While some specialists in internal medicine, particularly those working in cardiology, had attempted to develop objective criteria for making diagnoses, psychiatrists were the first to try to establish criteria on a large scale to define all the illnesses they treat.

The Washington University criteria for thirteen illnesses were published in 1972 in *Archives of General Psychiatry,* a widely circulated scientific journal. Although the criteria were developed for use in research, many psychiatrists in university medical centers found them useful for teaching medical students and psychiatric residents how to make psychiatric diagnoses. They also found them helpful in routine clinical evaluations of patients, since the criteria specified the information required to make a diagnosis and led to improved communication between clinicians and greater reliability.

In spite of their popularity in some scientifically oriented academic centers and their obvious usefulness, diagnostic criteria did not become familiar to most psychiatrists until quite recently. They might have remained in the hands of a few psychiatrists interested primarily in research were it not for a task force appointed by the American Psychiatric Association in 1974 to review and update the diagnostic handbook used by American psychiatrists, which went under the title of the *Diagnostic and Statistical Manual (DSM)*. Their work led to a dramatic revision of diagnostic procedures and practices in the third edition of the *DSM,* which finally appeared in 1980, known familiarly among psychiatrists as *DSM-III.* The most important of the many innovations contained in this new diagnostic manual was the enumeration of diagnostic criteria for the more than 100 disorders that it describes. Through this manual, one important aspect of the Neo-Kraepelinian revival—the emphasis on precise diagnosis based on careful study of objective symptoms—was officially mandated for all practicing psychiatrists. The Neo-Kraepelinian revival had become the *DSM-III* Revolution.

The DSM-III Revolution

The original *DSM-III* task force consisted of twelve people who met together in New York City in the fall of 1974. They were a group of psychiatrists and consultants from the fields of psychology and epidemiology who shared an interest in the process of making diagnoses and in methods for defining and classifying mental illnesses. Most were well-known researchers who had published widely in this area. In spite of this common interest, they differed in perspective and background, some with behavioral and psychodynamic orientations and some who were more biologically oriented Neo-Kraepelinians.

The night before that first meeting, these task-force members wondered what would happen the next day. Each had agreed to contribute voluntarily large amounts of time and energy to the process of developing a new *DSM*. Each had come hoping that his or her contribution would help improve the rather sorry state of the diagnostic process in psychiatry.

Robert Spitzer, the chairman of the task force, began the meeting by asking each of the new members to describe his or her background and to indicate the nature of the changes that he or she felt should be introduced into the new manual. One person began by lamenting the imprecision of psychiatric diagnosis and its poor reliability. He wondered if the new manual might not attempt to introduce more-objective definitions. Other members suggested that the new manual be based on research data rather than opinion, that the approaches used in the earlier manual *(DSM-II)* were clearly outmoded and often an embarrassment to the profession, and that perhaps the entire diagnostic manual should introduce specified criteria for each illness. When all the members of the task force had finished speaking, they were clearly astonished at the extent to which they agreed with one another. Each had come expecting to represent a minority point of view and to argue for increased objectivity and precision. Instead, each of the members was part of a unanimous majority. An era of opulent theorizing was passing into history. The members confronted their new task with an attitude that one called "dust bowl empiricism."

DSM-III was planned, written, field-tested, and reviewed by the American Psychiatric Association during the next six years. It was officially published in 1980. In a period when publishing in general has been a risky business, *DSM-III* became a best seller. Much to the surprise of the American Psychiatric Association, which was unprepared for the onslaught of orders, several hundred thousand copies were sold. Clearly, the new manual had something to say. What are the innovations that *DSM-III* has introduced? How has it changed the nature and process of psychiatric diagnosis?

THE INNOVATIONS OF *DSM-III*

DSM-III has led to a massive reorganization and modernization of psychiatric diagnosis. During the book's six years of development, the task force was expanded and many subcommittees appointed to study and define all types of psychiatric illnesses. The members of these subcommittees were leading experts in specific areas, such as anxiety disorders, schizophrenia, and the affective disorders. They were usually American, but occasionally experts from Great Britain were also consulted. In contrast to *DSM-II,* which was 119 pages long and enumerated only a few disorders, the new *DSM-III* is 494 pages long and describes over 100 disorders. Each disorder is discussed in extensive detail, drawing on all available research, and then defined with a specified set of diagnostic criteria. The nineteenth-century dichotomy between neurosis and psychosis was no longer used as an organizing principle. In early drafts, these terms were even deleted from the manual, but they were introduced in later versions because of an impassioned appeal from the more traditional forces in psychiatry.

Among these innovations, the introduction of diagnostic criteria has had the greatest impact. In order to appreciate the significance of this change, one must compare definitions in *DSM-II* and *DSM-III.* For example, manic-depressive psychosis, depressed type, is defined in *DSM-II* as follows:

> Manic-depressive psychosis, depressed type:
> This disorder consists exclusively of depressive episodes. These episodes are characterized by severely depressed mood and by mental and motor retardation progressing occasionally to stupor. Uneasiness, apprehension, perplexity and agitation may also be present. When illusions, hallucinations, and delusions (usually of guilt or of hypochondriacal or paranoid ideas) occur, they are attributable to the dominant mood disorder.

This description indicates some of the characteristics of serious depression, but it does not indicate how many of these must be present in order to be certain that the patient should definitely be given this diagnosis. Must the patient have all or only some? If only some, are some more important than others? How many symptoms are needed? All of us who have taken beginning psychology courses can appreciate how confusing such descriptions are. If quantitative and qualitative restrictions are not applied, then one can see oneself in almost every description of every illness. Thus the approach taken in *DSM-II* made the process of diagnosis inconsistent and imprecise.

The disorders described in *DSM-III* are defined very precisely. For example, the criteria for major depressive disorder (the disorder that corresponds most closely to the older manic-depressive psychosis, depressed type) can be paraphrased as follows:

Both of the Following Criteria Must Be Present:

I. A disturbance in mood characterized by depression, sadness, loss of interest or pleasure, or being "down in the dumps."

II. Persistence for a two-week period of at least four of the following symptoms:

1. Change in appetite or weight (poor appetite, weight loss, increased appetite, or weight gain).

2. Impaired sleeping patterns (either insomnia or sleeping excessively).

3. Objective evidence of either extreme restlessness or extreme decrease in motor activity.

4. Decreased interest or pleasure or decrease in sex drive.

5. Decreased energy or a tendency to tire easily.

6. Feelings of worthlessness, self-reproach, or excessive or inappropriate guilt.

7. Difficulty in thinking or concentrating.

8. Thoughts of death or suicide, or suicide attempts.

Additional exclusion criteria are also stated to rule out the possibility that these symptoms are due to a type of schizophrenia, organic mental disorder, or loss of a loved one.

A second innovation of *DSM-III* involved a thorough reorganization of the entire system for classifying disorders. *DSM-II* grouped disorders into just a few major categories: organic mental disorders, psychoses, neuroses, personality disorders, psychophysiological reactions, and disorders of childhood. This organizational system, as well as much of the older terminology, is modified in *DSM-III.* In recognition of the increasing awareness that there are many different discrete illnesses treated by psychiatrists, many more groupings have been introduced. The details of these changes are likely to be of interest only to psychiatrists, but a few instances are worth noting.

For example, the older term *manic-depressive psychosis* has been replaced by the term *bipolar disorder,* since the older term never made it clear whether the patient had both poles of the illness or only one.

The older term *hysterical neurosis* has been replaced by *somatization disorder* to eliminate the suggestion that this disorder could occur only in women. The use of the terms *neurosis* and *psychosis* has been minimized because these terms were used in so many different ways that their meaning was unclear. For example, the concept of neurosis has been variously used to refer to disorders characterized by psychodynamic conflict, disorders that produce psychological discomfort and are recognized by the self as uncomfortable (i.e., are "ego dystonic"), and disorders that are mild in comparison with the psychoses. The term *psychosis* has in the past been used to refer to disorders that are incapacitating, disorders characterized by loss of contact with reality, or disorders characterized by such symptoms as delusions or hallucinations. Because of their vagueness, both of these terms were dropped as organizing principles. The older psychoses and neuroses now appear under various headings and often with new names.

IMPLICATIONS OF THESE INNOVATIONS

As *DSM-III* was nearing publication, reports about it began to appear in the popular press. As might be expected, the document generated controversy both among psychiatrists and among their clientele. What are the implications of the changes introduced by *DSM-III?*

Perhaps the most important implication is a shift from a more psychoanalytic to a more medical approach. This shift is not obvious, but is suggested by a variety of subtle cues. One cue is a change in language. While *DSM-II* was not written for or by psychoanalysts only, it contained many terms frequently used by analysts, such as *impaired reality testing, conflict,* and *neurosis.* Most of this terminology has disappeared from *DSM-III* and has been replaced with terms that are more objective and descriptive. Opponents objected that the new language was dull, colorless, and dry. Proponents argued that the new language was clear, precise, and denotative. Behind the disagreement was a concern over the change in overall direction that these changes in vocabulary heralded. The new psychiatry was clearly moving back to an alliance with a mainstream medical tradition that emphasized the importance of careful definition of specific diseases based on *symptoms* rather than *dynamics.* Discussions of *DSM-III* in the lay press were often unfavorable, primarily because journalists (like most well-educated people) are drawn to the intricacies and complexities of psychoanalysis. They realized that a certain richness was symbolically lost in *DSM-III,* but did not appreciate the value of the objectivity that was also being gained.

A second implication of *DSM-III* affects the way psychiatrists evaluate and interview their patients. Ten or twenty years ago the patient who sought out psychiatric care was likely to receive (and also pay for) a relaxed and leisurely series of interviews. The doctor would ask the patient about a wide range of subjects in considerable detail, including early childhood experiences, his relationship with his parents, his relationship with his wife and children, his attitude toward his boss or his work, and his feelings about himself. Somewhere, embedded among these queries about personal and social aspects of his life, were questions about his symptoms. While psychoanalysts will no doubt continue to use this type of approach in spite of *DSM-III* (and indeed many of their concerns and techniques have little to do with the specific disorders described in *DSM-III),* the majority of psychiatrists are likely to focus on an evaluation of symptoms much more quickly. They will usually attempt to determine the patient's diagnosis during the first one-hour interview and will begin treatment, whether it be medication or psychotherapy, rather quickly after the first appointment. Whereas the older style of psychiatric interviewing used to stress the open-ended question and abundant use of noncommittal "uhs" and "ums," interviews based on a *DSM-III* approach are likely to be similar to those of internists or other doctors. The patient will be asked rather focused and detailed questions such as "How have you been sleeping?" "How has your appetite been?"

A third implication of *DSM-III* is that the diagnostic process has become clearer and more objective. The primary purpose of this change was to permit psychiatrists to communicate better with one another. By and large, this purpose has been fulfilled. A *DSM-III* diagnosis of major depressive disorder or schizophrenia has become much more standardized, so that clinicians in Peoria, Illinois, and White Plains, New York, can be more certain that they mean the same thing by these terms. An additional side effect, however, is that the diagnostic process has become demysticized, so that nonpsychiatrists can also understand what is going on. For example, lawyers can purchase *DSM-III* and use it to prepare for trials. They can quiz psychiatrists on whether or not the patient meets criteria for a given diagnosis. Insurance companies, such as Blue Cross/Blue Shield, can be more certain as to what a particular diagnosis means and whether treatment for that diagnosis is covered under a particular individual's policy. Patients who wish to claim they have a particular illness or attempt to obtain compensation for it can learn what symptoms they should describe simply for the price of *DSM-III.* To some, this demysticization of psychiatry is exciting and interesting, but to others (including insecure psychiatrists) it is frightening.

THE LIMITATIONS OF *DSM-III*

DSM-III has made, and will continue to make, many significant changes in the way psychiatrists think about and practice their specialty. But just as it is important to realize the changes that have been made, it is also important to realize the changes that have *not* been made. Two are quite important.

First of all, while *DSM-III* has moved toward the medical model, it has not embraced it wholeheartedly. What it shares with the medical model is an emphasis on the importance of diagnostic precision and careful delineation of the patient's symptoms. However, the medical model also assumes that a specific diagnosis ultimately defines a specific disease with a relatively discrete biological cause. *DSM-III* does not go that far. In fact, just as the words *psychosis* and *neurosis* are avoided, so, too, is the word *disease,* since it suggests a strong orientation toward the medical model. Each of the illnesses in *DSM-III* has carefully been named a disorder rather than a disease: major depressive disorder, somatization disorder, panic disorder, and so on from start to finish. Further, *DSM-III* attempts to maintain strict neutrality about the factors that may cause disease or disorder. As its preface points out quite rightly, we do not yet have definitive knowledge about the causes of most conditions that psychiatrists treat. Much research suggests biological causes for many of the major illnesses, but little is known as yet about the milder ones. Theories are abundant, but facts are few. Consequently, *DSM-III* avoids equally any discussion of psychodynamic theories, social theories, behavioral theories, or biological theories concerning the causes of illness.

A second limitation, and perhaps the most cogent criticism of *DSM-III,* is that it may gain reliability at the expense of validity.

Reliability refers to the *consistency* of a diagnostic system. If a system is highly reliable, then two different doctors are likely to come up with the same diagnosis after examining the same patient. Clearly, reliability is important. It is a necessary antecedent to validity, since clinicians who cannot agree about whether a condition is present or absent will certainly not be able to agree on anything else of importance. *Validity* refers to the *usefulness* of a diagnostic system. A diagnostic system that is valid helps the doctor to make predictions about important clinical aspects of the illness—what is causing it, what treatments are likely to be useful, whether the patient will recover, or whether the disorder can be communicated to others.

Unfortunately, the authors of *DSM-III* knew more about how to define disorders objectively than they did about these other important clinical aspects, primarily because psychiatry is still a young and intellectually growing specialty. For example, using *DSM-III,* psychiatrists are likely to agree reasonably well as to whether a given patient has a major depressive disorder. However, since this category is defined rather broadly and inclusively, some patients with this diagnosis are likely to respond to medications, while others might respond better to psychotherapy; some will recover fully, while others will not. Thus, this particular diagnosis, while it can be made reliably, cannot necessarily be used to make useful predictions about the future. This is, of course, a very important limitation.

In defense of *DSM-III,* it must be said that it has provided a necessary first step toward improving the validity of psychiatric diagnosis. Validity must be based on research, and research cannot be done unless disorders are defined reliably. The use of diagnostic criteria has already led to substantial improvements in psychiatric research, many of which are described in subsequent chapters. Even as they were writing *DSM-III,* its authors were concurring that it was a transitional document with many limitations. It was their fervent hope that *DSM-III* would quickly become obsolete and that during the coming years an improved *DSM-IV* would be developed that would be even more reliable and valid. The objective definitions of *DSM-III* are simply the first step in the biological revolution that is now occurring.

7

THE REVOLUTION IN DIAGNOSIS:

The Search for Laboratory Tests

Man, like any other thing organic or inorganic in the universe, grows beyond his work, walks up the stairs of his concepts, charges ahead of his accomplishments.

—JOHN STEINBECK,
The Grapes of Wrath

The process of going to see a doctor is only too familiar to most people: stopping at the front desk, being invited to take a seat in a crowded waiting room, spending half an hour reading outdated issues of magazines in which one has little interest, feeling flickers of anxious curiosity about whether the problem is "serious," and finally being ushered into a rather sterile examination room full of vinyl furniture with various kinds of equipment for taking blood pressure or looking into the eyes and ears. There is another fifteen-minute wait, this time without even the benefit of the dull magazine, during which anxiety mounts to uncomfortable proportions. Finally the doctor walks in the door, and the process of a diagnostic evaluation begins.

The specific details of any diagnostic evaluation vary, depending on the patient's problem and whether or not a specialist is being consulted. From a doctor's point of view, the components of the evaluation are the "history," physical examination, and laboratory tests. The doctor first inquires about the problems the patient has been having, which doctors usually refer to as the "chief complaint." After the patient states why he has come—an unexplained lump in his neck, soreness in his throat, or difficulty catching his breath when he walks up a flight of stairs—the doctor focuses on this particular problem and tries to figure out what is causing it. The doctor is taking a history of the present illness in order to be able to make a diagnosis. Being able to take a good history is considered the single most important skill in medicine. As he takes the patient's history, the doctor is trying to arrive at a "differential diagnosis," which is a list of the various diseases that might be causing the patient's chief complaint. Is the lump in the neck a swollen lymph node due to a streptococcal infection? Is it due to cancer? Is the shortness of breath due to pneumonia or heart disease? The doctor goes on to ask other questions that help him decide. "Have you been coughing?" "Have you been losing weight?" "Do you have any pain?"

By the time he finishes taking the history, the doctor is often fairly certain as to what is wrong with the patient. He then proceeds to do a physical examination, which will sometimes provide additional information, either confirming or disproving the probable diagnosis. Finally, after the physical examination, the doctor may decide to order some laboratory tests. These typically include various blood tests and/or X-rays. The choice of laboratory tests is closely tied to the provisional diagnosis. If pneumonia is a possibility, a chest X-ray is ordered. If there is no history of coughing, difficulty breathing, or chest pain, and if the physical examination shows no suggestion of fluid building up in the lungs, the doctor may decide not to order a chest film.

Until fairly recently, psychiatrists tended to use only part one of this three-part program of diagnosis. History-taking was all-important, while physical examination was likely to elicit few findings, and very few laboratory tests were available. In fact, traditional psychoanalysts refused to do physical examinations of their patients, since the intimacy of physical contact was likely to interfere with the psychoanalytic transference. If physical illness was thought to be a contributing cause of emotional problems, the patient was often referred to an internist or family doctor for further evaluation. Some psychiatrists, seeing themselves as examining the mind or brain, replace or supplement the physical examination with a "mental-status examination." This examination evaluates various mental functions, such as the ability to remember, to calculate, or to think abstractly.

As psychiatry is returning to a more medical orientation, however, psychiatrists are far more likely to perform physical examinations, particularly on patients admitted to the hospital or those patients who have some indication of a physical cause for their symptoms. Psychiatrists are also much more likely to order laboratory tests, such as routine blood work or chest films.

The most dramatic change that has occurred in the diagnostic process in psychiatry, however, has been the recent introduction of laboratory tests that may help illuminate the physical processes underlying the patient's symptoms. These tests are all relatively new, and none provides definitive proof of any particular diagnosis. Tests currently in use include a variety of techniques for brain imaging, the use of blood and urine measures of neuroendocrine and neurotransmitter function, and the use of the electroencephalogram (particularly during sleep) to evaluate the electrical activities of the brain.

Brain Imaging

Routine X-rays give beautiful pictures of very dense parts of the body, such as bone. They do not permit a doctor to see various organs within the body very clearly, unless the routine X-ray is supplemented by using some type of "radiopaque" substance that helps outline organs. Having a patient swallow barium in order to outline the esophagus, stomach, and intestines is an example of the latter. Since the brain is encased in bone, it is particularly difficult to see. Older X-ray techniques involved draining the cerebrospinal fluid from the ventricular system and injecting air into the ventricles, or injecting radiopaque substances into the arteries leading into the brain, but these techniques were painful and relatively risky. Consequently, they have been used only when a very serious physical illness, such as a stroke or a brain tumor, is considered highly likely.

Methods for seeing the brain in living human beings were revolutionized during the early 1970s through the introduction of a series of new "brain imaging" techniques. Unlike previous methods, most of these are relatively painless and harmless.

CT SCANNING

The most widely used technique for brain imaging is called computerized axial tomographic (CAT) scanning or computerized tomographic (CT) scanning. This technique, invented by Hounsfield of Great Britain in the early 1970s, involves sending an X-ray beam through a part of the body, such as the brain, to a set of detectors on the other side. Because the X-ray beam is diminished (or "attenuated") by the tissues it passes through, the information collected by the detectors on the other side can be used to construct a picture of different parts of the brain. Its various parts differ in density, with bone being most dense and fluids least dense. Table 4 summarizes the differences in density of various tissues in the brain, as measured by attenuation values or Hounsfield units, popularly known as "density numbers."

Table 4.
ATTENUATION VALUES OF
DIFFERENT TISSUES IN THE BRAIN

(Measured in Hounsfield Units)

Bone	+1000
Clotted blood	+ 95
Gray matter	+ 46
White matter	+ 32
Cerebrospinal fluid	+ 8
Fat	− 100
Air	−1000

The detectors break down the information they receive into a grid or matrix (80 × 80 units in early scanners, now as many as 320 × 320). Each position in this grid contains an attenuation number indicating the density of the particular small section of tissue in that grid, called a "volume element" or "voxel." The brain is also broken down into slices or cuts in order to improve the resolution of the image by making each voxel a relatively small chunk of tissue. Early scanners used a slice thickness of 13mm; more-recent scanners produce cuts as small as 2mm. In a scan consisting of 8mm slices and a 160 × 160 matrix, a voxel would represent a small block of tissue approximately 1.5 × 1.5 × 8mm.

The scanner eventually reconstructs a computerized image of the brain by rotating around the body one degree at a time and collecting more information on the detectors. This process continues until the scanning process has been completed for a full 360 degrees. In using density numbers to construct a picture of the brain, water is used as a reference point and assigned a value of zero. Various shades of gray, black, or white can then be assigned to the density number corresponding to each voxel. Cerebrospinal fluid, with a density similar to water, would appear to be nearly black, while bone would appear to be pure white. Gray matter would look lighter than white matter, since it contains less fat (the myelin sheath uses fat for insulation). A picture of the brain can then be constructed that is based on the shade of gray assigned to each tiny block of tissue.

A modern CT scanner gives a vivid picture of the brain. A clinician with a good knowledge of brain structure can look at a CT scan and mentally construct a three-dimensional picture of a given patient's brain. Figure 19 shows the relationship between standard CT scan slices and the various brain structures that can be seen on CT scans. Looking at the lowest levels, the clinician sees the cerebellum and the frontal lobes. Higher cuts pass through the frontal lobes and the language centers, while still higher cuts pass through the frontal, motor, and sensory cortex. The ventricular system, which stands out as a very dark region on the CT scan, assists in providing a clear landmark.

Figures 20, 21 and 22 show how vivid CT-scan pictures can be and indicate some of the information that clinicians can collect from CT scans. Figure 20 shows a CT scan from a normal sixty-year-old individual at a level corresponding to level 5 on the previous diagram. This level is also approximately the same as the section of the brain seen

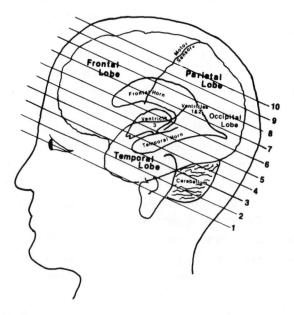

Fig. 19. **The relationship between CT scan cuts and brain structures.**

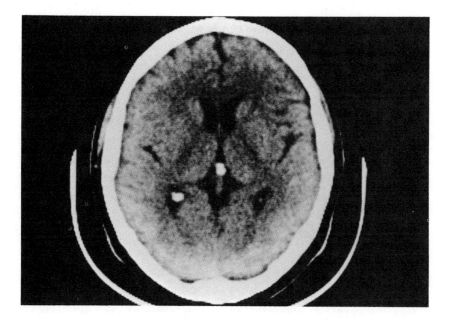

Fig. 20. Normal CT scan.

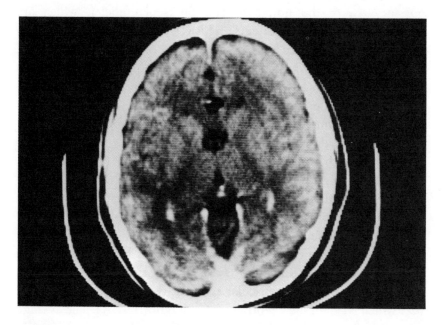

Fig. 21. Abnormal CT scan of a schizophrenic patient showing enlargement of the limbic system and a lipoma of the corpus callosum.

in figure 3 of chapter 5. If one compares the structures seen in figure 3 with those seen in the CT scan, it is evident that a good modern scanner can delineate gray and white matter quite clearly. (Remember that on CT scans the shades of gray are reversed, and that gray matter apears lighter than white matter.) In this scan one can see the large thalami on either side of the third ventricle, the caudate nucleus lying just beneath the frontal horns of the two lateral ventricles, and even the rest of the striatum. The bulk of the brain appears relatively darker in comparison with these lighter regions of gray matter. One can also see a hint of the pale rim of cortex around the edge. The white area in the center is a calcified pineal gland, and calcifications are also seen in the venous tissue inside the posterior horn of the left lateral ventricle. (Such calcifications are common and do not imply disease.)

Figure 21 is a scan of a patient suffering from schizophrenic symptoms and shows structures found at the same level. This patient has a very abnormal CT scan. The pitch-black substance seen in the center is a lipoma (or nonmalignant fatty tumor) that lies on top of his corpus callosum. In the region where his frontal horns should be, he instead has three peculiar-looking fluid-filled spaces. These lie below an important area of the limbic system, the septal nuclei, which are markedly enlarged. Higher cuts on his CT scan show that the lipoma is a large structure that runs along the top of his corpus callosum, which is markedly thickened and enlarged. The patient suffers from severe delusions that have not improved in spite of rigorous treatment. These various structural brain abnormalities may account for his schizophrenic symptoms and their poor response to treatment.

The abnormalities seen in figure 21 are relatively unusual. Figure 22 shows a much more common abnormality observed in schizophrenic patients. This CT scan shows two cuts from the brain of a twenty-eight-year-old man who had symptoms similar to those of Roger Wallis, the patient with chronic symptoms of schizophrenia described in chapter 4. The first cut is at approximately level 7; it shows the high ventricular region. The ventricles in this man's brain are relatively enlarged for his age. Radiologists and psychiatrists have developed a method of measuring ventricular size that corrects for overall brain size, which is called the "ventricular-brain ratio" (VBR). The average ventricular-brain ratio in a normal individual of this age is about 4.5. This man's VBR is about 12, a significant enlargement. Further, a

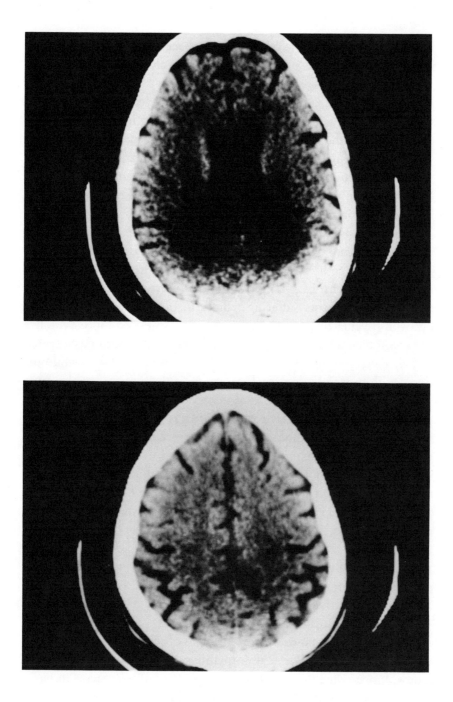

Fig. 22. Abnormal CT scan of a schizophrenic patient. Above, ventricular enlargement. Below, cortical atrophy.

higher cut shows the cortical sulci that are seen when one looks at the top of the brain. These sulci are also markedly enlarged.

Both these findings indicate that the patient's brain has shrunk and withered. In short, although only twenty-eight years old, this patient has brain abnormalities similar to those observed in people suffering from severe dementia or people of extreme old age. These types of CT-scan abnormalities, particularly ventricular enlargement, are relatively common in patients suffering from schizophrenia. John Hinckley, the young man who attempted to assassinate President Reagan, had very similar abnormalities on his CT scan.

Psychiatrists are still exploring the significance of these various types of CT-scan abnormalities observed in schizophrenia. Early reports aroused the hope that CT scanning might provide a "laboratory test" for schizophrenia—that is, CT-scan abnormalities would be present in most patients suffering from schizophrenia, and would not occur in psychiatric patients with other diagnoses. As more evidence has accumulated during the past several years, it has become clear that not all schizophrenic patients have CT-scan abnormalities, while patients with other illnesses, such as mania or dementia, may also have abnormal CT scans. Thus, CT scanning does not provide a true diagnostic laboratory test, but it does provide a large amount of significant information about pathological processes occurring in the brains of schizophrenic patients.

The scan shown in figure 21 helps confirm that some types of schizophrenia may be due to abnormalities in the limbic system. The patient whose scan appears in figure 22, showing marked ventricular enlargement and cortical atrophy, had a different set of symptoms and perhaps a different underlying pathological process. While the first patient suffered primarily from delusions of persecution, the second patient had more prominent "negative symptoms," such as avolition, alogia, and affective flattening.

One of the most exciting areas of current research in psychiatry involves attempting to relate various types of schizophrenic symptoms to various types of CT-scan abnormalities, in the hope of developing a new, more refined classification system. If schizophrenia is in fact a group of two or more different types of diseases, then each might have different symptoms and different causes. For example, the patient whose scan showed the lipoma, who suffers from persecutory delusions, might have an abnormality in his limbic system leading to excessive dopaminergic transmission; alternatively, his callosal thickening might reflect excessive electrical activity and communication going on between his two hemispheres, making him oversensitive to events occurring around him and eventually leading to suspiciousness, irritability, and feelings of persecution. On the other hand, the other patient with an abnormal scan has an illness quite similar to dementia. In fact, he has Kraepelin's dementia praecox. Further, he has a brain similar to that noted in people with dementia. His symptoms, such as inability to think clearly or loss of interest in his surroundings, are also not unlike those of demented people. In his case, the search for causes will focus on something likely to produce diffuse brain damage, such as a viral illness early in life causing brain inflammation and leading to later brain atrophy.

Thus many psychiatrists have begun to order CT scans frequently for those patients in whom the diagnosis of schizophrenia or dementia is likely. Many of these patients will have completely normal CT scans, but some will have abnormalities of the type shown in figures 21 and 22. When these abnormalities are noted, they indicate that the patient's symptoms are probably due to a structural cause in the brain. Since ventricular enlargement is relatively common in schizophrenia, this finding may also help confirm the diagnosis of schizophrenia. John Hinckley's abnormal CT scan suggests quite strongly that he suffers from schizophrenia: Behind his abnormal behavior is an abnormal brain.

When structural brain abnormalities are noted in patients suffering from schizophrenia, the result may suggest something about how they should be treated. Rather sadly, some of these patients do not respond as well to neuroleptic drugs as do patients with normal brain structure. Because schizophrenia is such a handicapping disease, most psychiatrists will nevertheless choose to treat patients with ventricular enlargement with medication, at least initially. If the patient shows a poor response, the psychiatrist may eventually discontinue the drugs or prescribe only low doses, inferring that the abnormalities in the structure of the brain cannot be modified by a chemical method. Thus CT scanning is not only useful in understanding the nature of the patient's symptoms and their underlying pathological process in the brain, but may also assist in predicting and understanding the response (or lack thereof) to treatment.

CT scanning has been in existence for only ten years and has been used in psychiatry for an even shorter period of time. Structural brain abnormalities in schizophrenia were first reported by Johnstone and Crow of Great Britain in the *Lancet* in 1976. While the original findings have now been widely repeated in many different centers throughout the world, scientists are still trying to determine the types of abnormalities occurring, the extent to which they are more characteristic of schizophrenia than other types of mental illness, and the best ways to develop objective measures from CT scans. Older scanners had relatively poor resolution and did not give good pictures of small brain structures, such as the caudate or the thalamus. Research in the future is likely to capitalize on the improved precision of the new high-resolution scanners in order to determine whether particular parts of the brain are selectively atrophied. Some preliminary reports suggest that frontal regions of the brain may have a greater degree of atrophy, particularly on the left side. Investigators are just beginning to use the actual density numbers to study the brain, rather than relying on the pictures that are produced from them. As techniques for analyzing CT scans improve in scientific sophistication, CT-scan research promises even more interesting and exciting results during the next five to ten years.

NUCLEAR MAGNETIC RESPONSE (NMR)

Nuclear magnetic response (NMR) is a technique that is just beginning to enjoy wide use and which promises to yield a great deal of information in the future. It has two main advantages over CT scanning. First of all, it produces images of extremely high resolution. Structures in the brain can be seen in incredibly fine detail, with very clear differentiation between small gray and white-matter structures. For example, it is difficult to see the mammillary bodies on CT scan, but they can be seen clearly using NMR. The second advantage is that NMR achieves these pictures of living tissue at essentially no risk. Unlike CT scanning, which uses a small amount of radiation, NMR uses none.

The NMR scanner produces images by capitalizing on the fact that our body cells are rich in hydrogen, phosphorous, and other elements that are sensitive to electromagnetic forces. NMR scanning is done by placing the patient inside a huge circular magnet. The electromagnetic forces produced by this magnet cause the hydrogen atoms in the body to move in response. When the force is then turned off, they move back to their original position, in the process producing an electromagnetic signal. Different tissues in the body produce different signals, depending on the mixture of elements they contain. As in the case of CT scanning, these signals can be fed into a computer and turned into tiny dots of black, shades of gray, and white, which then create a picture of body tissues. While CT-scan cuts tend to be fixed at relatively arbitrary points, the NMR scanner can produce pictures that slice through the head in any direction and at any angle, providing many more different views of the three-dimensional structure of the brain.

At the moment, NMR is in use at only a few medical centers throughout the country. During the next ten years, it will no doubt become as widely used as CT scanning has been during the previous ten years. It is too new to have been used in any detailed quantitative research in psychiatric patients, but these studies are just now beginning. They should be watched with interest, since they are likely to yield even more precise information about the nature of brain abnormalities in mental illness than has CT scanning.

REGIONAL CEREBRAL BLOOD FLOW

CT and NMR scanning give what is known as a "static" image of the brain; hence they can be used to look for abnormalities only in brain *structure*. During recent years, investigators have also been working to develop techniques of "dynamic" brain imaging. A dynamic approach permits one to actually observe how the brain works when it performs certain tasks. In other words, it provides a way of measuring *function* rather than *structure*.

The two commonest techniques for dynamic brain imaging are studies of regional cerebral blood flow (RCBF) and positron-emission tomographic (PET) scanning (discussed below). Both of these techniques are at present highly experimental and are used primarily for research, but the study of regional cerebral blood flow may become a common clinical tool during the next few years.

The technique of RCBF involves the use of radioactive tracers, principally xenon-133, which are taken up in brain tissue and can be used to visualize which parts of the brain are most active. In early RCBF studies, xenon-133 was injected into a blood vessel. Recently, however, the technique has been refined so that the patient need only inhale xenon-133, which then accumulates in the brain. The labeled xenon emits photons, which can be measured either by mapping flow on the surface of the brain or with a computer-assisted tomograph much like that used in CT scanning. At the present time, however, the resolution of tomographic RCBF is much poorer. In current use, pictures are obtained of three cross-sectional brain slices that are 4cm apart. Since many important structures in the brain—such as portions of the ventricular system or the basal ganglia—are only about a centimeter in size, current methods for measuring RCBF do not permit a detailed visualization of deep brain structure. The surface, or cortical, maps are more accurate, but do not permit examination of deep brain structure.

Figure 23 shows the three cuts that are used at present in tomographic RCBF studies, depicting the brain of a "normal" individual. (It happens to belong to the author of this book.) Slice 1 passes through the cerebellum, the temporal lobes, and the lower frontal lobes; it corresponds roughly to slices 3 and 4 in figure 19. Slice 2

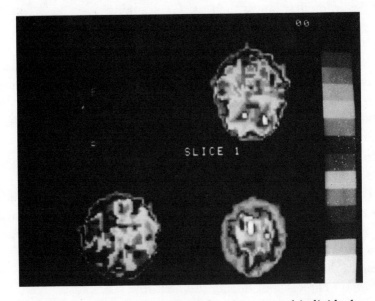

Fig. 23. Regional cerebral blood flow in a normal individual.

(lower left) passes through the occipital lobes, the superior temporal lobes and language regions, and the frontal lobe; it corresponds roughly to slices 5 and 6 in figure 19. The highest cut (lower right) passes through the parietal, motor, and frontal regions and corresponds to slices 7, 8, and 9 in figure 19.

In normal individuals, the lower cuts have a characteristic pattern, which appears in brilliantly colored images—an example of which appears on the dust jacket. Cut 1 is an "ace of spades," while cut 2 is a "Maltese cross." These patterns, which are more difficult to see in black and white rendering, are produced by assigning colors on the basis of the number of photons emitted from the xenon taken into the brain. Regions where blood flow is very high, reflecting a high level of brain activity, emit more photons and are assigned brighter colors, such as shades of red. "Cold" areas, where less activity is occurring, are assigned blues and greens. This normal scan, done while the patient is resting but with eyes open, shows hot areas in the cerebellum on the lower cut and hot areas in both temporal lobes and the midfrontal and occipital regions on the second cut.

Research with RCBF is still in its infancy. Only a few centers in the United States have facilities for measuring RCBF, and research in these centers is only beginning. The technique can be used to study regional blood flow in various types of diseases. In patients who have had strokes, for example, blood flow will be reduced in damaged parts of the brain. It can also be used to determine whether patients suffering from particular kinds of mental illness have greater or lesser blood flow in particular areas of the brain than do normal people.

Figure 24 shows the results of one investigation of RCBF in mental illness. Researchers at Southwestern University in Dallas have completed a study comparing regional blood flow in patients suffering from depression during the course of treatment. The figure shows blood flow in two different patients. Both show similar changes after treatment. In both photographs the center cut is shown at three different times. The first picture shows the RCBF pattern before treatment. The scan has a characteristic patchy "moth-eaten" appearance with many blue and green (pale gray) areas of low blood flow. As treatment progresses, perfusion clearly increases. The second picture is brighter, and the third brighter still. Pictures of this type suggest that patients suffering from depression may have a decreased metabolic rate in their brains, which may be either a cause or a symptom

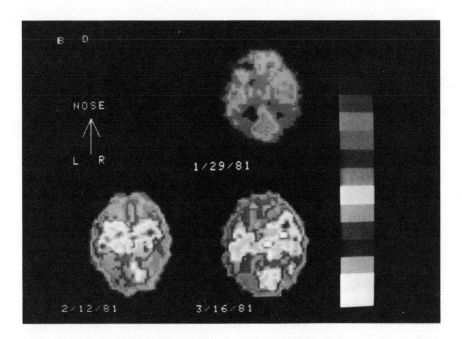

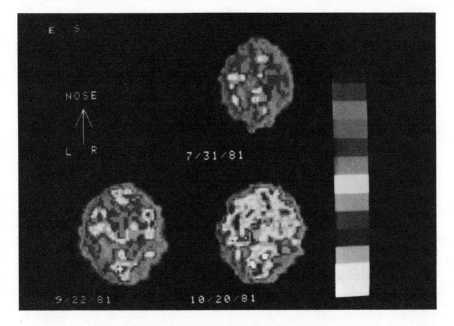

Fig. 24. Regional cerebral blood flow in depression.

of the disease. In any case, when the depression goes away with treatment, the metabolic rate (as reflected by cerebral blood flow) goes up. Thus, one application of this technique may be to monitor response to treatment.

PET SCANNING

PET scanning is a technique that combines the best of both worlds. It gives good resolution, much like CT scanning, permitting the clinician to see brain structures in relatively fine detail. Further, like RCBF, it is a dynamic technique that permits the neuroscientist to watch the brain at work and to observe which parts of it become more active in response to various kinds of stimuli. Thus PET scanning is a wonderfully exciting technique that may assist in unlocking many of the secrets of schizophrenia and other major mental illnesses during the next few years.

Unfortunately, however, PET scanning also has a number of drawbacks. Most important, it is at present a *very* expensive technique, and likely to remain so for some time. While the cost of a CT scan or an RCBF study is in the neighborhood of several hundred dollars, the cost of a PET scan is measured in thousands of dollars. Further, unlike CT scanning or RCBF, it does carry some risk. The only risk in CT scanning is a very modest amount of radiation exposure, about equal to that of a routine chest X-ray. RCBF, although it involves the inhalation of a radioactive substance, xenon-133, also carries a low risk, again about the same amount of radiation as a chest X-ray. In CT scanning, the principal site receiving radiation is the brain, which is not at all sensitive to radiation, while in RCBF the radiation exposure is to the throat and lungs, which are somewhat more radiosensitive. Moreover, the patient receiving a CT scan or RCBF study experiences no subjective discomfort, whereas PET scanning requires the injection of radioisotopes into a blood vessel, entailing a small amount of subjective pain as well as a small additional risk.

PET scanning works in a manner similar to RCBF and CT scanning. Radioactive substances are introduced, taken up in the brain, and radiation is then emitted from those parts of the brain that are most active and therefore take up the largest amounts of the isotope. Information about the amount of radiation taken up is collected on a set of detectors surrounding the brain in a 360-degree circle. As in CT scanning, the brain is broken down into relatively small grids and sectioned in slices. While PET scanners can potentially "see" structures as thin as 1 to 2 millimeters, scanners currently do not yield such fine resolution.

PET scanning is expensive because it is at present the ultimate high-technology brain-imaging technique. While RCBF studies use relatively stable radioactive tracers, PET uses unstable substances that are positron-emitting—hence the name "positron-emission tomography," or PET. PET scanning requires a team consisting of physicists, neurochemists, engineers, and medical clinicians. The physicists and engineers must create the positron-emitting isotopes, which are produced in a cyclotron that must be located adjacent to the PET-scanning site, since these isotopes begin to decay quickly and are only useful for minutes to hours. The cyclotron must be encased within huge walls of cement in order to protect the nearby environment from radiation risk. Within the cyclotron, protons are accelerated and bombard substances commonly found in the body, such as oxygen or nitrogen, turning them into positron emitters. Chemists must quickly attach these radioactive positrons to a molecule that is frequently used in the brain, such as glucose. This chemical substance is then injected into a patient's artery by a team of clinicians, and the activity of the brain can then be measured.

During the past several years, PET scanning has been used to study brain function in patients suffering from affective illness, schizophrenia, and childhood autism. The technique has usually involved injecting glucose labeled with the fluorine-18 positron. Since glucose (or sugar) is the fuel that provides brain cells with nourishment to carry on their activities, it serves as a useful substance for seeing which parts of the brain are most active metabolically. To date, most studies have been done with the subject simply lying at rest and thinking about whatever she chooses. Normal people who do this tend to have the greatest activity in their frontal lobes—or a "hyperfrontal" pattern, whereas patients suffering from autism and schizophrenia may have a "hypofrontal" pattern while at rest. There is also a suggestion that the decrease in activity may be greater on the left side of the brain than on the right.

PET scanning is a technique whose story will evolve in many different directions during the next ten years. Because the technique is so complicated and so expensive, it will probably never be used frequently for clinical evaluation or screening as CT scanning is now and NMR or RCBF may be during the next few years. On the other hand, PET scanning *will* be used in elegantly designed research investigations of the major mental illnesses. Neuroscientists are still trying to figure out the best way to gain the maximum amount of information from this exquisite technology. In particular, clinicians are trying to decide the best types of subjects to study. Should we focus on patients with prominent negative symptoms? Should we try to find out whether positive symptoms reflect abnormal activity in some specific part of the brain, such as the auditory or language centers? Should we try to study patients both at rest and when they perform tasks that require activation of a particular part of the brain, such as speaking or reading, in order to determine whether patients with mental illnesses have a particular kind of deficit?

Further, neurochemists are working to develop new ways to label substances that may provide interesting clues about "chemical breaks" in the brain. For example, in the future almost certainly positron-emitters will be attached to psychoactive drugs or known neurotransmitter substances and their activities traced in the brains of patients with mental illness, thereby helping us map areas of drug action and of abnormalities in neurochemical transmission.

Neurochemical Tests

X-ray techniques, such as the brain-imaging techniques just described, permit one to actually see inside the body. For the clinician and neuroscientist eager to understand what is happening in the brains of their patients, the chance to look inside the skull without causing any physical discomfort to the patient is as intriguing and exciting as an array of holiday gifts is to a ten-year-old child.

Neurochemical research, while equally exciting, is several steps farther from reality. Rather than permitting direct visualization of what is happening inside the brain or body, neurochemical research tends to proceed by inference. Samples of blood or urine are collected and then studied to determine whether they contain unusually large or small amounts of chemicals known to occur in the brain or known to affect people's emotional and mental condition. Many different types of laboratory tests of blood and urine are currently being examined and developed experimentally. Several have already proved so useful that many psychiatrists obtain them relatively routinely in patients with significant or severe symptoms. In particular, these tests tend to be widely used in patients suffering from depression.

TESTS OF NEUROENDOCRINE FUNCTION

Thoughtful doctors have noticed for many years that patients suffering from depression have many symptoms similar to those occurring in people with diseases of the thyroid or adrenal glands, two important glands that regulate body function. The thyroid is located in the neck, just below the "Adam's apple," and controls or modulates body temperature, heart rate, and other aspects of metabolic function. The adrenal glands are located on top of the kidneys (*ad-renal* = above the kidneys); they modulate our body's capacity to respond to various stresses by producing the substance known in medicine as "cortisol," which is familiar to lay people as cortisone. When these glands are not working properly, patients have symptoms such as fatigue, change in appetite, or insomnia, all of which are also common symptoms of depression.

Although these glands are located outside the brain, they are controlled by it, as we saw in chapter 5. The command center for neuroendocrine control resides in the hypothalamus and the pituitary. As seen in chapter 5, the hypothalamus has many connections with the limbic system and the rest of the brain. Figure 25 shows in schematic form how the brain regulates and modulates neuroendocrine function, using the adrenal glands as an example.

When we are confronted by a major stress, which may be psychological (as when a loved one dies) or physical (as when we are in an automobile accident), this information is perceived and felt by our brains. Recognizing that we will need extra resources of energy and alertness to cope with the stress, the brain sends a message to the hypothalamus telling it to stimulate the pituitary to release more cortisol, the major hormone that the body uses to confront stress. The messenger used by the hypothalamus to "talk" to the pituitary is a peptide hormone, corticotropin-releasing factor (CRF), while the messenger from the pituitary to the adrenals is adrenocorticotropic hormone (ACTH). The adrenals then pour out cortisol, and informa-

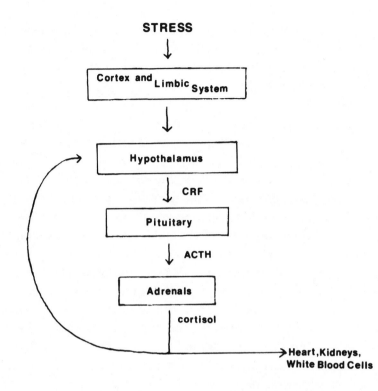

Fig. 25. Hypothalamic regulation of the adrenal system.

tion about the amount of cortisol in the bloodstream is sent back to the hypothalamus, which is sensitive to plasma cortisol levels. If the hypothalamus senses that these need to be even higher, it sends out more CRF. On the other hand, if the hypothalamus senses that circulating cortisol is high enough or too high, it stops sending out CRF. Thus the whole system is regulated by a set of feedback loops, which of course are somewhat more complicated than portrayed in this schematic diagram.

The suspicion that patients suffering from depression might have neuroendocrine abnormalities, particularly abnormalities of cortisol production, has been confirmed by a series of studies conducted during recent years. The earliest research demonstrated that some patients suffering from depression produced abnormally large amounts of cortisol, although it was not clear whether this was a cause or an effect of the illness. In order to explore the mechanism that might be involved, during the mid-1970s research psychiatrists began to experiment with a laboratory test frequently used in internal medicine to evaluate patients suffering from Cushing's disease, an illness characterized by excessive cortisol secretion from the adrenals. This test is called the "dexamethasone-suppression test" (DST). Psychiatrists soon learned that the DST could also tell them something about patients suffering from depression. It has now become a common laboratory test used to evaluate patients suffering from depression.

The DST is specifically designed to determine where the communication system between the brain and the adrenal glands has broken down. It works by having the patient take a tablet containing dexamethasone, a potent synthetic hormone very similar to cortisol. As the dexamethasone circulates in the blood and travels up to the brain, the hypothalamus in normal individuals "reads" plasma cortisol levels as being high because it interprets the dexamethasone as equivalent to cortisol. It stops sending out CRF to the pituitary, and in turn the pituitary stops sending out ACTH to the adrenals. Thus, taking the dexamethasone tablet "suppresses" the hypothalamic-pituitary-adrenal axis, and within twelve hours the blood levels of cortisol drop to low levels. This is known as "normal suppression."

Many patients with depressive illnesses fail to suppress in this normal pattern; something has gone wrong in the hypothalamic-pituitary-adrenal communication system, and cortisol continues to pour out. Even though the patient has taken dexamethasone the night before in order to "fool" the hypothalamus, when blood samples are taken the next morning and in the middle of the next afternoon or evening, plasma cortisol levels continue to be high. Thus the patient's DST is said to be "abnormal."

The DST is important not only because it helps illuminate neuroendocrine abnormalities in depression but also because it is sometimes used to help diagnose depression. Investigators in a number of different research centers have now documented that among psychiatric patients abnormal DSTs occur most frequently in patients hospitalized for depressive illness. When patients with other types of psychiatric problems, such as schizophrenia or panic disorder, are tested, most of them suppress normally. Only about half of the patients with major depression have abnormal DSTs, however, and since so many patients with well-defined depressive illness have normal DSTs, it is not a perfect "laboratory test" for depression. Still, it is often useful to clinicians in clarifying the diagnosis when there is a difficult differential diagnosis—for example, between schizophrenia and a depression with many psychotic features. The DST is also helpful because it tends to return to normal when the patient has recovered from depression, and thus it provides a useful method of monitoring response to treatment.

The significance of the high rate of abnormal DSTs in patients suffering from major depression is still unclear. It does seem to suggest that part of the cause of the illness may reside in the brain, particularly the hypothalamus or the higher brain centers that govern it. In order to explore the precise nature of this "nervous breakdown" in more detail, researchers are now investigating how the hypothalamus and its target organs respond to other neuroendocrine "challenge tests," such as those developed to explore hypothalamic-pituitary-thyroid function. These tests, however, are at present much more experimental than the DST. As the results of this research unfold in the next five to ten years, we hope to have a much more precise notion of the mechanisms that underlie depressive illness.

MHPG EXCRETION

Another laboratory test that is enjoying increasingly wide use in psychiatry is the evaluation of MHPG excretion. MHPG (shorthand for 3-methoxy-4-hydroxy-phenylethyleneglycol) is an important breakdown product of norepinephrine, one of the major transmitters in the central nervous system. As we shall see in more detail in chapter 9, the most widely accepted theory about the cause of depression is the "catecholamine hypothesis." This hypothesis suggests that patients suffering from depression have a deficit of norepinephrine in the brain, leading to a generalized slowing and impairment of function that expresses itself as depressive symptoms. A great deal of research during the past decade has been devoted to determining whether the catecholamine hypothesis is correct. As is often the case in medical research, particularly that involving human beings, the answer is both yes and no—but perhaps "yes" more than "no."

In studying the norepinephrine system in depression, one tactic that has proved particularly useful has been to measure the amount of MHPG excreted in the urine. When this was done, it turned out that some patients had relatively high MHPG, some low MHPG, and some an intermediate level. Investigators then began to examine how the three different groups of patients with depression might differ in other important ways. They soon noted that the three groups tended to respond to *different* types of antidepressant medication. Those patients with low MHPG tended to respond best to antidepressant drugs that appeared to stimulate the norepinephrine system in the brain, while those with high MHPG tended to respond better to antidepressant drugs that affect the serotonin system.

Although this test of neurotransmitter function has not yet explained the mechanism causing depression, it has provided doctors with some clinically useful information about selecting a particular type of medication for a particular patient. It suggests that there may be several different kinds of abnormalities in neurotransmitter function in depression. Those patients with low norepinephrine and low MHPG should perhaps be placed on one particular class of drugs, while patients with high MHPG should be given an entirely different drug. These results explain why not all patients put on antidepressants uniformly do better (although many do). As tests like this are refined and used more widely in the future, they may become standard ones that clinicians obtain before prescribing medication for their patients.

The Electrical Activity of the Brain

As we saw in chapter 5, the brain is a mass of electrical circuits that continuously fire messages back and forth between various control centers in the brain. Just as we have learned to "see" the brain through brain imaging, or to make inferences about its control over the rest of the body through measuring chemical by-products, so too we can study what is happening inside people's skulls by measuring the electrical activity of the brain.

The technique of electroencephalography (EEG), the measurement of "brain waves," was developed by Hans Berger in the 1930s. EEG is a relatively painless and simple laboratory test whose workings are quite similar to those of the more familiar electrocardiogram used to monitor cardiac function. As in an electrocardiogram, small metal disks, called "electrodes," are placed on the skin (over the chest for an EKG and on the scalp for an EEG) using a salty jelly that aids the transmission of electrical impulses. The electrodes are attached by wires to a recording device, which then produces a series of squiggly lines reflecting the electrical activity of the area being measured. As in the EKG, a large amount of additional information can be obtained by comparing electrical activity between different electrodes that are wired together in a standard pattern. The electrodes are spread across the scalp so that the activity in all regions—including frontal, temporal, parietal, and occipital—can be measured.

Over the years, investigators have succeeded in mapping the patterns of brain waves that tend to occur in normal people when they are awake and when they sleep. For example, the electrical activity in the frontal region is usually relatively faster—a rhythm of about twenty cycles per second that is called "beta rhythm." The electrical activity seen over the occipital region is typically slower, approximately eight to twelve cycles per second, and is called "alpha rhythm." When we become drowsy, the electrical activity of our brains slows down to four to eight cycles per second, called "theta rhythm." When we fall deeply asleep, brain activity slows down to three to four cycles per second, "delta rhythm."

Because the EEG measures electrical activity only on the surface of the brain, and because it summarizes the electrical activity of billions of neurons, it provides only a crude measure of brain function. Until relatively recently, its chief application in psychiatry has been to rule out various neurological diseases that may masquerade as psychiatric disease.

For example, patients with epilepsy have seizures because a particular part of their brains is overexcitable and prone to fire in a wild or uncontrolled manner, sometimes setting off the electrical "explosions" that produce grand mal seizures, or seizures of other types. When the EEG of an epileptic patient is recorded, small spikes are usually noted in the region of the brain that is overly excitable; these spikes are particularly likely to appear when the patient becomes drowsy or falls asleep.

Patients with the type of epilepsy involving the temporal region, called "psychomotor epilepsy" or "temporal lobe epilepsy," are prone to have symptoms similar to those observed in some psychiatric illnesses. Especially when the abnormal focus is on the left side, patients with temporal lobe epilepsy tend to be obsessional, humorless, very concerned with religious ideas, and to have little interest in sex

—not unlike some patients with obsessive-compulsive personality. Other patients with psychomotor epilepsy are prone to occasional outbursts of violence or dissociativelike episodes. Still others may have periods when they have psychotic symptoms. Sometimes these symptoms can be diminished by treatment with antiepileptic drugs, and so it has been important to psychiatrists for many years to rule out epilepsy, particularly temporal lobe epilepsy, as a cause of such symptoms.

More rarely, psychiatric symptoms may also be caused by brain tumors. Since the invention of the CT scan, these are best diagnosed through brain-imaging techniques. Prior to CT scanning, however, the EEG provided a useful screening test for brain tumors.

During the past twenty years neuroscientists have begun to focus specifically on the electrical activity of the brain during sleep. Through this research, they have discovered that during a normal night's sleep, people pass through a series of characteristic stages. These are summarized in figure 26, which portrays the electrical activity of the brain during an eight-hour period. The EEG while awake is predominantly beta activity—a fast, low-voltage activity. Thereafter, our brains pass through four characteristic stages of sleep. While we are in these stages, our sleep is further divided depending on whether we are dreaming or not dreaming. When we dream, our eyes become very active, moving back and forth and generating large bursts of electrical activity, which is called REM (rapid eye movement) sleep. We tend to have short periods of REM sleep interspersed throughout the night. The bulk of our brain activity while sleeping,

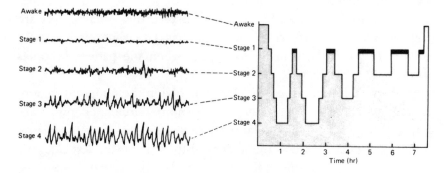

Fig. 26. Stages of sleep.

however, is in a non-REM pattern. In figure 26, the periods of REM sleep are characterized by dark bars.

During Stage 1, our normal waking brain activity begins to slow down. During Stage 2, little bursts of symmetrical waves, called "sleep spindles," appear, indicating that we are becoming very drowsy and falling asleep. During Stage 3 sleep, we fall into a theta pattern, and during Stage 4 sleep we pass into a delta pattern. We remain in Stage 4 for the first sixty to ninety minutes of sleep, then cycle back to Stage 1 and have a short burst of REM sleep during which we dream. Then we cycle down into deep Stage 4 sleep again for another hour or so, moving back up again to a somewhat longer period of REM sleep in about the third hour. As the pattern continues on, later in the night we have less delta and more REM sleep.

Perhaps the commonest complaint in psychiatric patients, particularly those suffering from depression, is insomnia. Consequently, during recent years investigators have become interested in examining the EEG patterns of such people when they are sleeping. Not surprisingly, they have noted that depressed patients tend to have abnormal EEG patterns during sleep. In particular, these patients tend to move very rapidly into the first period of REM sleep. Whereas a normal person spends about ninety minutes sleeping before the first REM period, patients suffering from depression sleep for only about forty minutes before the first REM period. Sleep researchers call this "decreased REM latency." Patients suffering from depression also tend to have increased REM density, or longer periods of REM sleep, than do normals. Finally, they also tend to have less delta sleep and a shorter period of sleep.

These laboratory studies of sleep in depression confirm that the depressed patient's subjective complaint of insomnia is supported by objective research indicating that indeed the sleep patterns *are* disturbed—the depressed patient usually does not sleep as deeply or as long. They also imply yet again that something has gone wrong with the brain's regulatory mechanisms in people suffering from depression.

Some psychiatrists believe the sleep EEG is an additional laboratory test that can be used to assist in the diagnosis of depression. Depending on how decreased REM latency or other abnormalities are defined, approximately 70–80 percent of patients suffering from depression have abnormalities in their sleep EEGs.

Although it is painless, the sleep EEG is a relatively time-consuming and elaborate "laboratory test." At the moment, it is used in only a limited number of centers throughout the country, although its clinical applications do appear to be broadening. Within a few years, more clinicians may be ordering sleep EEGs as an additional aid in making a diagnosis. Even if the sleep EEG does not become widely accepted as a clinical laboratory test, it has served as another useful research tool. Like the other laboratory tests we have examined, the sleep EEG points yet again to the brain as the place where a "break" has occurred in patients suffering from depression.

8

THE REVOLUTION IN TREATMENT:

The Search for Somatic Therapies

Much Madness is Divinest Sense—
To a discerning Eye—
Much Sense—starkest Madness—
'Tis the Majority
In this, as All prevails—
Assent—and you are sane—
Demur—and you're straightway dangerous—
And handled with a chain.

—EMILY DICKINSON,
No. 435

Figure 27 shows the "tranquilizing chair" invented by Benjamin Rush. As described earlier, Rush was an eighteenth-century Philadelphia physician who took a special interest in mental illness, wrote the first American textbook of psychiatry, and cared for the mentally ill who were admitted to Pennsylvania Hospital, which was founded in 1751 by Benjamin Franklin and was the first hospital built in the United States. Viewed from the vantage point of the late twentieth century, Rush's tranquilizing chair seems to contradict his humanitarian ideals. The chair was a treatment developed to calm agitated patients. They were strapped in by all four extremities with their eyes and ears covered, remaining there until they became calm.

In Rush's "modern" psychiatric wards, the mentally ill were not chained to walls (as they still often were in Europe), but were allowed to walk freely and to lead as normal a life as possible. Nevertheless, patients sometimes became physically violent, making them dangerous to themselves or to others. In these circumstances, some type of treatment was required. The tranquilizing chair was the best that one of the most enlightened minds in a relatively enlightened era could come up with. Rather worse versions of the tranquilizing chair were developed by other people in other places at other times. For exam-

189

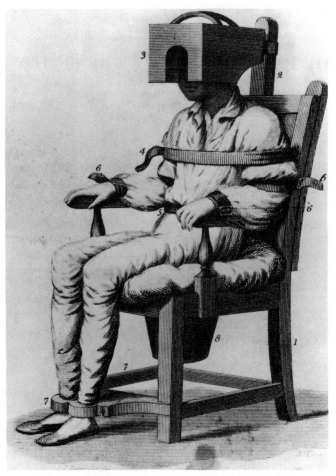

Fig. 27. Benjamin Rush's "tranquilizing chair".

ple, the "Darwin chair," created a few years later by Erasmus Darwin (grandfather of Charles), was a chair in which agitated psychotic patients were strapped down and then whirled around rapidly; the treatment was considered complete when blood emerged from their ears. Straitjackets were the twentieth-century equivalent of these older treatments.

The paraphernalia of physical restraints have all but disappeared from the modern psychiatric hospital during recent years, an innovation made possible by the biological revolution in psychiatry. Physical restraints have become outmoded and unnecessary because they have been replaced by a wide range of medications and other treatments that have been discovered during the past thirty years and that have dramatically changed the treatment and outcome of the major mental illnesses. These treatments are called "somatic therapies" since they act on the brain, which is part of the *soma* (body), while the psychotherapies by contrast are thought to act on the *psyche* (mind). (Ultimately, the psychotherapies must also act on the brain, since that is where the mind resides, but we are still far from understanding how or why.)

Unlike the tranquilizing chair or the straitjacket, which only controlled and protected the patient, the new somatic therapies are genuine *treatments*—they actually eradicate many of the symptoms of mental illness, perhaps by correcting an underlying neurochemical abnormality. The discovery of these treatments has revolutionized the care of the mentally ill as much as the discovery of penicillin and insulin has changed the care of people suffering from infections or diabetes. "Wonder drugs" are now available to diminish the symptoms of three out of four of the major categories of mental illness: affective disorders, schizophrenia, and anxiety disorders. Now that we have discovered that the effects of these illnesses can be reduced through modulating brain chemistry, investigators are continuing to search for even better treatments, and they are still at work attempting to find a treatment for dementia.

The Earliest Discovery: Paris, 1952

The first powerful drug available to treat serious mental illness was discovered in much the same way as was penicillin: by accident. The discovery was the happy consequence of a chance finding being observed by a person with a fertile mind who could recognize its larger implications.

The story begins with the development of the antihistamines during the 1940s. Histamine is a chemical that occurs naturally in the body and is released when our bodies encounter something to which they are allergic, producing the familiar symptoms of watering eyes, running nose, swelling, redness, and itchiness. The antihistamines block the effects of histamine and thus can be used to relieve people of the discomforts of allergic reactions (such as hay fever). During the 1940s, many physicians recognized that antihistamines might also have other useful properties. In particular, surgeons were interested in using them to prevent surgical shock (a serious drop in blood pressure during surgery), since histamine release was known to trigger a reduction in blood pressure.

A French surgeon, Henri Laborit, is recognized as the major pioneer in developing the new drugs that would eventually revolutionize psychiatry. He gave his patients an antihistaminic phenothiazine, promethazine, which is still widely used in the United States under the name Phenergan. Although it did not have the expected effect of preventing a drop in blood pressure, Laborit noticed that it did have other desirable effects. Patients who took it became somewhat sleepy and markedly less anxious, but were still clearly aware of everything going on around them and able to communicate. These effects could also be observed after the surgery. Laborit reported: "Even after major operations they are never excited, do not complain, and genuinely appear to suffer less." Thus phenothiazine medications were introduced as an important preoperative treatment prior to general anesthesia, a use they still enjoy today.

Laborit's report triggered a search for new and better drugs that might be even more useful. Such research tends to be strictly empirical —that is, chemists tinker around with the structure of the original parent compound, adding a chlorine atom here or a methyl group there, and then test the new compound to see if it has different effects in laboratory animals and eventually in human beings. One drug, to which a chlorine atom was added (and which therefore was called "chlorpromazine"), seemed to work particularly well in animals. When Laborit then tried it in his patients, he discovered that it had marvelously calming effects on them preoperatively, even better than promethazine. The patients were conscious, aware of everything going on around them, mildly drowsy, but above all tranquil about the prospects of surgery. This led Laborit to wonder whether the drug might be useful in psychiatry.

The first experiments with chlorpromazine (Thorazine) in psychiatric patients were completed in Paris in 1952 by two French psychiatrists, Jean Delay and Pierre Deniker. They gave this new medication to patients with many different types of illness, including mania, depression, and schizophrenia. It soon became clear that the drug had powerful calming effects on agitated psychotic patients, producing the same mixture of tranquilization and mental alertness that it had in the preoperative patients. Much more exciting, however, was the discovery that this new drug was especially effective in patients suffering from schizophrenia. Not only were agitated schizophrenics calmed, but the new drug seemed to eradicate or markedly diminish the terrifying hallucinations and troubling delusional thoughts that occur so frequently in schizophrenic patients. In short, the drug did more than just tranquilize, although that was an obvious and important effect. It also appeared to have very special ameliorative effects on the major psychotic symptoms, such as delusions and hallucinations. For the first time in the history of psychiatry, a drug had been found that could be used to treat these devastating symptoms. Patients who had been ill for some time often showed striking improvement, and young patients who had become ill only recently seemed to return to normal after treatment with chlorpromazine. For the first time in many years, patients, families, and doctors were able to feel hopeful.

The results in Paris were confirmed all over the world in the next several years. Within a very short time, chlorpromazine became the established treatment for schizophrenia. Patients who had been unable to live outside a hospital sometimes improved so much that they could leave and live on their own. Over the course of the next twenty years, the number of patients in mental hospitals in the United States dropped by about 50 percent. For those patients who remained in the hospitals, the atmosphere had changed: Even though they were not well enough to leave, they often improved enough to lead more normal, albeit restricted, lives—playing games, participating in activities outside the hospital such as excursions to movies or to go shopping, and staying in touch with the outside world through magazines, newspapers, and television. The occasional patient who was unpredictably violent, and therefore dangerous to himself and to other patients on the ward, could now be calmed quickly through medication. The feared straitjacket disappeared, taking its place alongside the tranquilizing chair in the historical museum of antiquated treatment methods.

The Search Continues

One "wonder drug" might seem quite enough, but for various reasons clinicians and researchers quickly began to search for other, even better medications. One factor was the problem of "side effects." Most drugs have both "target effects" and "side effects." The target effects act on the major symptoms of a particular illness—the accumulation of bacteria in the case of penicillin, or the presence of delusions and hallucinations in the case of schizophrenia. Along with these desirable effects, however, drugs also have side effects that may be undesirable, such as indigestion or diarrhea in the case of some antibiotics. Chlorpromazine sometimes produced drowsiness or a diminution of alertness, troublesome side effects for the patient who wished to drive a car or return to school. In addition, chlorpromazine sometimes produced symptoms similar to those occurring in Parkinson's disease—rigidity, tremor, a shuffling gait, and immobility of facial expression. Chemists in the pharmaceutical laboratories hoped that by modifying the chlorpromazine molecule, they might be able to retain more target effects and eliminate some of the unwanted side effects. Their efforts were further spurred when it became obvious that chlorpromazine would have a large market. Since it was a patented drug, only one company could produce and market it, but other pharmaceutical companies could get on the economic bandwagon by marketing a drug with similar effects but a slightly different structure and a different name.

During subsequent years, many other medications cascaded from the pharmaceutical industry. To the extent that the lay public could follow these changes at all, they were puzzled by the large variety of different names and different drugs that promised new and better results. (Adding to the confusion is the fact that every drug has both a generic [chemical] name and a trade name. Chlorpromazine, for example, is the generic name, while Thorazine is the trade name under which this drug was marketed. When a company's patent on a drug expires, as it does after twenty years, the drug can be marketed by other companies under a new trade name.) Inadvertently, however, the process of searching for new antipsychotic medications led to another very exciting discovery.

Not long after chlorpromazine appeared, the Swiss pharmaceutical firm CIBA Geigy tinkered with it and produced a new substance that they called "imipramine" (Tofranil is the trade name). Animal research indicated that the drug seemed harmless and had quieting effects much like chlorpromazine. The drug was given to a Swiss psychiatrist, Roland Kuhn, so that he could determine how well it worked on schizophrenic patients. Kuhn found that it had very little effect on delusions and hallucinations, but he noted that the drug seemed to relieve depressive symptoms. Experiments with other patients suffering primarily from depression indicated that indeed imipramine, a drug only slightly different from chlorpromazine, had specific effects in relieving depressive symptoms. In fact, it produced many remarkable cures.

Thus, another new class of drugs had been created almost overnight: the tricyclic antidepressants. As figure 28 indicates, the tricyclic antidepressants are very similar in structure to antipsychotic agents such as chlorpromazine. The removal of a sulfur atom at the top of the center ring and a chlorine atom on the right creates a drug that has extraordinarily different effects on target symptoms. (As that figure also indicates, a drug such as chlorpromazine also has a "tricyclic" structure in that it is composed of three circular benzene rings. Nevertheless, by convention, clinicians refer only to the tricyclic antidepressants as "tricyclics.")

The subsequent story of imipramine and other tricyclics is quite similar to the story of chlorpromazine. Investigators in Europe discovered that the drug was remarkably effective in lifting patients out of severe depressions: People who had been ill for some time recovered quite miraculously. The drug quickly spread to the United States, and by the mid- to late 1950s it was widely used both for outpatients and for hospitalized patients who were suffering from serious depressive illness. Other pharmaceutical companies made minor modifications and produced "me too" tricyclic antidepressants such as amitriptyline

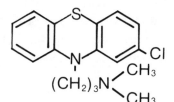

Chlorpromazine
(The first neuroleptic)

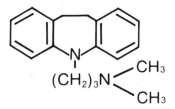

Imipramine
(The first antidepressant)

Fig. 28. Structural similarities of chlorpromazine and imipramine.

(Elavil) or desipramine (Norpramin). While initially it seemed that these drugs differed primarily in their side effects (some were more sedating than others), recent evidence suggests that they may also have differential effects on the noradrenergic versus the serotonin systems in the brain. (More about that later in this chapter and in chapter 9.)

About the same time that the tricyclics were being discovered, another class of drugs for treating depression appeared as well. These are the "monoamine-oxidase inhibitors" (MAOIs). Again, a drug developed for other purposes was recognized by astute clinicians to have significant effects on the symptoms of mental illness. In this case, the drug was iproniazid, an antibiotic developed for treatment of tuberculosis. Some of the tubercular patients were quite depressed; and yet when they were given iproniazid, their depressive symptoms appeared to improve. This observation led to the familiar pattern of trying the drug in a relatively broad range of psychiatric patients, noticing that it worked particularly well for depressive illness, and thereafter using it as a relatively specific treatment for a particular type of mental illness. Iproniazid itself is no longer widely used, for it has been succeeded by other, more effective MAOIs such as Nardil and Parnate.

Another new class of drugs introduced in the heady atmosphere of the 1950s included the antianxiety agents or "minor tranquilizers," the earliest of which was meprobamate (Miltown). Prior to their introduction, the barbiturates (such as phenobarbital or amobarbital) were sometimes used to treat the symptoms of anxiety. They were far from satisfactory, however, because they were originally meant to be "sleeping pills" and thus often led to marked sedation. In addition, they tended to produce "tolerance"—that is, over a period of time, larger and larger doses were needed to produce the same effect. The barbiturates are also habit-forming, so excessive use of phenobarbital to treat anxiety could lead to addiction.

The new antianxiety drugs seemed at first to eliminate many of these problems. The original prototype, meprobamate, was eventually found to have some undesirable properties, such as excessive dependence and a high lethality rate when taken in suicide attempts. The next generation of antianxiety drugs, the best known of which are Librium and Valium, have become household words and are perhaps the most widely prescribed drugs in the United States.

Because drugs like Thorazine and Valium were introduced at more or less the same time and were both called "tranquilizers," people have sometimes failed to realize how different they are. Pharmacologists and psychiatrists originally divided these two groups of drugs into "major tranquilizers" and "minor tranquilizers." The major tranquilizers, such as Thorazine, were used for the more incapacitating mental illnesses that tended to be characterized by psychotic symptoms such as delusions and hallucinations. The minor tranquilizers were used to relieve the "nervousness" that accompanies the anxiety disorders. These two groups of drugs thus act on quite different target symptoms, although they share the common property of "tranquilizing" or calming.

Unfortunately, sometimes even doctors did not always understand that the drugs acted on quite different target symptoms and instead assumed that if a "minor" tranquilizer was effective in relieving anxiety, then a "major" tranquilizer might be even more effective. This sometimes led to the inappropriate use of drugs such as Thorazine for the treatment of anxiety disorders, causing unwanted side effects and inadequate relief of anxiety. Further, while the schizophrenias are usually more incapacitating (and therefore more serious) than the anxiety disorders, anyone who suffers from a severe anxiety disorder will testify that her illness should hardly be considered a "minor" one that can be treated with a "minor" class of drugs. Thus the term *tranquilizer* has been largely dropped by physicians who are knowledgeable and up-to-date, although they may still sometimes use this term because it is more familiar to the lay public. The proper terms for the class of drugs to which Thorazine belongs are the "antipsychotics" or the "neuroleptics" (nerve modulators), terms that describe the actual target actions of the drugs. Medications such as Valium or Librium are now called "antianxiety agents."

By the end of the 1950s, the basics of modern psychopharmacology had been developed and established. In the 1960s only one more major drug was added to the therapeutic armamentarium. This drug was lithium carbonate (or lithium chloride in the earliest trials). Lithium chloride is a naturally occurring salt, analogous to the sodium chloride that we all use to salt our food. In fact, its first use in medicine was as a salt substitute for people suffering from hypertension who needed a low-sodium diet. It was soon discovered, however, that high doses of lithium carbonate tended to make people sick, and so lithium was abandoned as a salt substitute. In the late 1940s, the Australian John Cade was using lithium in experiments with guinea pigs and noticed that they seemed sedated by it. He then tried the drug on agitated psychotic patients and found it to be quite useful. Nevertheless, lithium was slow to catch on initially because of its bad reputation as a salt substitute.

During the 1960s most of the fundamental work on the usefulness of lithium in mania was completed by Mogens Schou and his collaborators in Denmark. Like Cade, Schou found that lithium calmed agitated patients and was particularly effective in people suffering from mania. Chlorpromazine was effective as well, but it had unwanted side effects such as lowering of blood pressure, dry mouth, and "Parkinsonian" or "extrapyramidal" side effects such as tremor and rigidity, whereas lithium had almost no side effects when administered in small doses. Manics who had been sleepless, overactive, and garrulous were calmed and returned to normal within a few weeks. Furthermore, in a carefully designed longitudinal study, Schou also observed that patients placed on maintenance lithium tended to have a much lower rate of recurrence than did patients who did not receive maintenance lithium. Thus the drug not only relieved the target symptoms of mania but also seemed to have a prophylactic (preventive) effect. Some evidence suggested that it normalized or stabilized mood so well that patients often lost the tendency to swing low into depression and high into mania. By the early 1970s, a large mass of evidence had been accumulated, all of it indicating that lithium was a powerful and effective drug for the treatment of affective disorders. Thus in 1970 the Food and Drug Administration (FDA) granted doctors permission to prescribe lithium for mania in the United States.

How Are Drugs Tested?

The development and introduction of new drugs is carefully controlled in the United States by the FDA and carefully monitored by the scientific community. As the previous accounts indicate, drugs are usually tried first in animals to ensure that they produce no harm in addition to certain desirable effects. Nevertheless, there are no mental illnesses in animals that are closely equivalent to the mental illnesses that devastate human beings. Therefore, the usefulness of a new drug can be established only through clinical trials in human beings suffering from particular types of mental illness.

While early trials of a new drug may simply involve giving it to patients and seeing if their target symptoms improve (an "open trial"), the most rigorous and definitive test of any new medication is the "double-blind trial." In a double-blind trial, a new drug is matched against one or two other drugs. The other drug may be a placebo that has no recognized therapeutic effectiveness. In a more rigorous trial, the comparison drug is one with known therapeutic effectiveness; it serves as a standard against which the new drug may be measured to determine whether it is equally effective or even more so. In such trials neither the doctor nor the patient knows which person is receiving which drug—both are blind, hence the trial is termed "double-blind."

In a well-designed trial of this type, the new drug and the comparison drug are packaged identically. In addition, if a placebo is used, it may be modified in some way so that it produces side effects similar to those of the new experimental drug. The patient is told in advance that he may be receiving an experimental drug and signs a form indicating that he has consented to participate in a clinical experiment. The doctor and patient observe and rate the course of his symptoms. After a set period of time, the code is broken and the investigators find out if the new drug is effective.

This type of rigorous trial is needed because of the well-known "placebo effect"—that is, many patients tend to get better just because *something* has been prescribed for them. A placebo (the word means "I shall please") is a substance with no known therapeutic effect. A substantial number of patients given placebos by a doctor report that they feel better. Some of this improvement may be due to the power of suggestion: People who think they are being helped somehow convince themselves subjectively that improvement has occurred. Some patients may get better because the natural course of the illness is short-lived and episodic. The common cold, for example, usually lasts only about a week. It is caused by viruses rather than bacteria, and yet many patients are given prescriptions for antibiotics (which kill bacteria but not viruses) and report experiencing substantial relief from this medication. They do not realize that their symptoms would have gotten better anyway, because the natural history of the common cold is short-lived and episodic.

The drugs used in modern psychiatry have all passed the stringent test of a double-blind trial. They have been proved to be more effective than placebos, and the newer ones are at least as effective as the older ones such as chlorpromazine or imipramine. In spite of this rigorous test, new drugs have proliferated in all major classes, so that psychiatrists now have available many different types of drugs in the three major classes just described: antipsychotics, antidepressants, and antianxiety agents. The remainder of this chapter summarizes the way these various types of drugs are used in modern psychiatry and some of the consequences of this revolution in treatment that has occurred in the past thirty years. It provides an overview of all types of somatic therapy used to treat the four major classes of mental illness: affective disorders, schizophrenias, anxiety disorders, and dementias.

Treatment of the Affective Disorders

The two poles of the affective disorders, mania and depression, have quite different symptoms and demand quite different types of treatment.

TREATMENT OF MANIA

The treatment of mania usually involves one or more types of somatic therapy: lithium carbonate, neuroleptics, and (rarely) electroconvulsive therapy (ECT). Lithium is the preferred treatment and is usually used first. If it is successful in curing the mania, lithium alone will continue to be used. Neuroleptics may be added if the patient's symptoms are resistant to treatment, and ECT is used very infrequently for those patients who do not respond to either lithium or neuroleptics. ECT is also used occasionally during the first trimester for pregnant women suffering from mania whose unborn children might be harmed by lithium.

Lithium is present in the human body in trace amounts. Sodium, a nearby salt on the periodic table, is present in the body in much larger amounts. As we saw in chapter 5, sodium, together with potassium and calcium, regulates electrical conduction in our nerve cells. Sodium is the positive ion that moves into the nerve cell and permits positive electrical charges to flow through it. While we do not yet know precisely how lithium works to relieve the symptoms of mania, one mechanism of action could be its effect on the electrical conduction of nerve cells.

Patients suffering from mania usually require hospitalization, which may last from a week to one or even several months. Lithium is often prescribed initially in a dose of approximately 1800mg. Within several days after the medication is begun, the level of the drug in the bloodstream has stabilized and can be monitored by drawing small amounts of blood and measuring the lithium level. Doctors usually try to maintain a level of around 1.0 (measured in milliequivalents of lithium per liter of blood), although the level may be allowed to go somewhat higher in patients who are seriously agitated and psychotic. It is necessary to monitor blood levels, since lithium can have toxic effects if the level is allowed to go too high. In simple, straightforward cases, the manic symptoms go away within a few days to a week or two, and the patient is returned to her normal self. The transformation often seems quite miraculous.

After the manic symptoms have disappeared, the dose of lithium is usually reduced to about half of the earlier therapeutic dose. The patient is kept on this maintenance dose of lithium, which typically ranges from 900 to 1200mg, as an outpatient. As we saw in chapter 4, mania is a disease that tends to recur. Consequently, doctors have to leave patients on maintenance doses of lithium for extended periods of time, and perhaps for a lifetime. Patients sometimes try to experiment with discontinuing the drug on their own. Unfortunately, all too frequently this leads to another attack of mania, which may require another hospitalization and disruption of a patient's work and personal life. Eventually most patients who experiment in this way accept the fact that taking medication daily is a small price to pay for peace of mind.

The side effects of lithium are minimal. Some patients experience a metallic taste, hand tremor, nausea or other indications of stomach upset, or feelings of sluggishness. Since lithium can produce stomach irritation, it usually should be taken with meals or with a glass of milk. If the blood level of lithium becomes too high, patients may experience symptoms of toxicity, which include mental confusion, feelings of extreme heaviness in the arms and legs, and vomiting and diarrhea.

These symptoms usually indicate that a blood level should be obtained and that the medication should probably be temporarily discontinued.

Long-term risks of drugs are always a source of concern to both doctors and patients, especially for drugs that may be needed for many years. Although lithium has been certified for use in the United States by the FDA only since the early 1970s, patients in Europe and Australia have taken it for as long as thirty years. Most have had no problems, but in a few patients long-term complications have been observed. The two most important complications involve the thyroid gland and the kidneys. A few patients treated with lithium for many years have developed goiter or thyroid insufficiency, which leads to inadequate production of thyroid hormone. This problem is easily treated through taking thyroid hormone orally to correct the deficiency. A rarer complication is cellular changes in the kidneys, which is potentially a much more serious long-term effect. As yet it is not clear that this problem occurs with significant frequency or even that it is definitely due to lithium therapy. Nevertheless, because of these potential long-term hazards, every doctor and every patient must weigh the potential risks against the potential benefits of long-term lithium use.

This dry recounting of dosages and side effects does not do justice to the enormous impact that lithium has had on the lives of patients suffering from mania. When they are not suffering from an episode of mania, patients with bipolar affective disorder are often very talented, creative, and highly successful people. Their episodes of mania can disrupt and even devastate their lives. A costly high flight into mania is often followed by a downward crash into depression. Lithium tends to truncate both the highs and lows, normalizing mood in people who felt otherwise condemned to cycle helplessly up and down, never able to achieve a golden mean. As stated earlier, well-known creative individuals such as Robert Lowell have suffered from bipolar disorder. When lithium became available to American psychiatrists during the early 1970s, these individuals gave testimony to its effectiveness in normalizing their lives and enhancing their creative powers.

Neuroleptics are the other group of medications used to treat mania. Before lithium was available, neuroleptics were the treatment of choice. They continue to be effective medications for the treatment of very severe mania that cannot be controlled by lithium alone. Typically, they are used during the first or second week of a manic attack, and often tapered and discontinued when the lithium begins to take hold. The neuroleptics used most frequently include Thorazine and Haldol. Since these drugs are used most often to treat schizophrenia, their complications and side effects are discussed in the section on the treatment of schizophrenia.

Very infrequently, ECT is used as a treatment for mania. Prior to the development of lithium and neuroleptics, it was the only effective treatment available and was used quite often. Now it is used only for the occasional patient who does not respond to medication or for the rare patient to whom medication might pose some risk, such as a woman during the first three months of pregnancy. Since ECT is used much more often as a treatment for depression, its nature and complications are described in the following section.

TREATMENT OF DEPRESSION

Depressive illness does not always require treatment with somatic therapy. Sometimes people experience a full depressive syndrome, as defined by a standard diagnostic system such as the *DSM-III* criteria described in chapter 6, and yet the depressive episode is short-lived, clears spontaneously, or responds to several sessions of talking with a therapist or counselor. It would be wasteful and expensive to treat these mild, brief depressions with medication.

Ever since antidepressant medications became available, psychiatrists have devoted considerable time and effort to determining how to predict which patients are most likely to need somatic therapy. One widely used distinction is between "endogenous" and "reactive" depression (or "melancholic" versus "nonmelancholic" depression in more recent terminology). Endogenous or melancholic depression is more severe and more likely to require some type of somatic therapy. The older term *endogenous* implies that the depression "grows from within" or is biologically caused, with the implication that unfortunate and painful events such as losing a job or a lover cannot be considered contributing causes. On the other hand, "reactive" depression by definition is the type that follows such unfortunate events. Thus the older terminology highlights the importance of precipitants in a person's private life and seems to imply that depressions occurring after misfortune have no physical component and are not likely to respond to somatic therapy.

That is simply untrue. A more modern point of view recognizes an interaction between a person's life situation and his body's reaction to it. Depression is one such reaction. Thus the terms *endogenous* and *reactive* are gradually being abandoned because they are misleading. Nevertheless, psychiatrists tend to cling to old terminology, and many continue to use the term *endogenous* even though they do not necessarily mean that a person with endogenous depression is free from recent painful experiences that might serve as contributing causes. They use other important characteristics to identify an endogenous or melancholic depression in order to decide whether or not to prescribe medications.

First of all, they examine the patient's symptoms. Patients with a medication-responsive depression tend to have many "vegetative" or physical symptoms, such as insomnia, loss of appetite, weight loss, diminished sex drive, or diurnal variation. Psychiatrists also examine specific aspects of the patient's change in mood. If the mood is "non-reactive," so that the person is unable to brighten up when something pleasant occurs, this is further evidence that the person is endogenous or melancholic.

They also examine clues from the patient's history. If relatives have had problems with affective disorder, this also suggests a genetic or biological component. If the patient has had previous episodes of depression, evidence is piled even higher, and the evidence is especially strong if the patient has responded well to somatic therapy in the past.

Further, a doctor looks at the effects of the depression on the patient's life. If the depression is so severe that it is incapacitating, so that the person is unable to work or manage routine daily life, this also suggests the possible need for medication. Mary Williams, the patient described in chapter 4, had many of these classic features suggestive of an endogenous or melancholic depression that is likely to respond well to medication.

Finally, the doctor may order laboratory tests, such as the dexamethasone-suppression test or a sleep EEG, in order to assist in her decision about prescribing medication. She will also try to determine whether the patient has seriously considered suicide. If so, she may well decide to hospitalize the patient in addition to prescribing somatic therapy.

Three somatic therapies are used for the treatment of depression: tricyclic antidepressants, monoamine-oxidase inhibitors (MAOIs), and electroconvulsive therapy (ECT).

Many different tricyclic antidepressants are currently available. Some of the most widely used include imipramine (Tofranil), amitriptyline (Elavil), desipramine (Norpramin), nortriptyline (Aventyl), and doxepin (Sinequan). More recently, a new group of "second generation" antidepressants has been developed. These new antidepressants have a four-ring rather than a three-ring structure and are therefore referred to as "tetracyclics." The antidepressant drugs all seem about equally effective in reducing depressive symptoms when they are tried on large groups of depressed patients. Any one of them is effective about 70 percent of the time.

Why then does a doctor choose one drug instead of another? One reason is that while all are about equally effective in achieving *target effects,* such as relieving low mood or loss of interest, they differ significantly in their *side effects.* One important way in which they differ is in the amount of sedation that they produce. The tricyclic antidepressants can be placed on a continuum, with Norpramin being least sedating, Elavil and Sinequan most sedating, and Tofranil and Aventyl somewhere in the middle. Doctors often try to capitalize on these side effects to help relieve a patient of some of her more troubling symptoms. For example, if agitation and insomnia are important complaints, a doctor may select a more sedating antidepressant such as Elavil. On the other hand, if a patient complains of extreme lethargy, a doctor may select a more energizing antidepressant such as Norpramin.

These drugs may also differ in terms of the neurotransmitter systems that they act on. While there is some overlap, Tofranil and Norpramin appear to act on the noradrenergic systems in the brain, while Elavil seems to act on both the noradrenergic and the serotonin systems. There may well be several different types of depressive illnesses due to different underlying abnormalities in brain neurotransmitter systems. If so, this explains why some patients respond better to a particular drug such as Elavil while others respond better to Tofranil. One suffers from a serotonin deficiency in the brain, while the other suffers from a norepinephrine deficiency. Thus it is reasonable to switch from one type of antidepressant to another if the patient does not respond adequately.

While the antidepressants are genuine "wonder drugs," they are not without their problems. They are relatively slow to act, often requiring two to three weeks in order to reduce target symptoms sufficiently so that the patient feels "back to normal." Many patients take these drugs expecting to feel better within a few days, and they are disappointed to find that the "wonder cure" does not begin immediately. Indeed, because of problems with side effects, some patients even feel quite a bit worse for the first few days. In addition to the sedation that occurs with some antidepressant drugs, most produce a few other unpleasant effects, such as dry mouth, tremors, blurred vision, bloating and weight gain, urinary retention, or light-headedness on standing up suddenly. Patients should be warned about these unpleasant side effects so that they do not feel tempted to discontinue the medication before it takes effect.

Dosages of tricyclics vary depending on the particular drug. For most, the dose usually ranges from 100 to 200mg. Many psychiatrists consider that a particular medication has not been given a fair test unless the patient has taken it in a dose of at least 150mg for at least three weeks. (A few antidepressants such as Aventyl are prescribed in much smaller doses because they carry more potency per milligram. Knowing exactly what the dose should be for each drug requires medical training and experience. The doses mentioned in this chapter are intended as rough guidelines and should not be taken as rules.) Some doctors have access to laboratories that can be used to monitor blood levels to make sure that the patient is on an adequate dose. Unfortunately, however, much of the necessary basic research has not yet been done in order to establish the best blood level to get the best therapeutic response.

The tricyclics are powerful drugs for treating depression. Some patients feel their symptoms lift slowly and steadily over the course of days to weeks, while others report a change almost overnight after several weeks on the medication. In addition to being wonder drugs, however, they are also dangerous drugs. Since patients suffering from depression are at high risk for suicide, and since tricyclics can be lethal when taken as a suicide attempt, depressed patients for whom tricyclics are prescribed should be observed closely by their family members and their doctors. Sometimes doctors will give patients only enough drugs to last for a few days or a week in order to minimize the risk of overdose. These drugs should also not be left around where small children may be able to get hold of them.

Because many types of tricyclics are available and most are quite effective, the MAOIs (e.g., Nardil, Parnate) are used relatively infrequently. They tend to be used in those patients who have tried a wide range of tricyclics and have not responded. The MAOIs are second-choice drugs because they have many more complications and side effects than do the tricyclics. In particular, the MAOIs can interact with a wide variety of popular foods to produce a dangerous and potentially life-threatening rapid rise in blood pressure. The foods that must be avoided by anyone taking MAOIs include red wine; beer; cheddar and other aged cheeses; chocolate; chicken livers; coffee; and a variety of pickled and salted foods, such as soy sauce, sauerkraut, and salted or pickled fish. While many people could give up chicken livers or pickled herring without discomfort, living without red wine, beer, chocolate, and coffee condemns one to a rather austere existence. Nevertheless, the MAOIs work well for a few patients.

ECT is another treatment sometimes used for depression instead of tricyclics. ECT has been used for many years and is well recognized as one of the most effective treatments available for depression. Nevertheless, it has received a very bad press, and many people fear it. Films like *One Flew over the Cuckoo's Nest* have portrayed ECT quite inappropriately as a form of punishment used to control disruptive patients. In the early days when ECT was first introduced, it was often given without adequate sedation beforehand and without the use of muscle relaxants to prevent violent seizures; in such cases the treatment *was* both frightening and risky.

Modern ECT is a different matter. Just prior to the actual treatment, the patient is given a dose of a short-acting barbiturate that puts him to sleep. He is then given a powerful muscle relaxant that prevents his muscles from contracting violently when the convulsion is induced. The actual seizure is produced by placing two electrodes just above the patient's temples (sometimes only one, on the right side) and passing a very small amount of electricity through the brain. This current activates the brain and produces a seizurelike activity, manifested by jagged spikes on an EEG monitor. The patient's body is relaxed, however, and shows no signs of a seizure because of the muscle relaxant that he has been given earlier. The seizure is over in about a minute and the patient wakes up soon thereafter. Patients suffering from depression are usually given approximately eight treatments, although some receive as few as three or four and others require as many as twelve to fifteen. The treatments are usually given every other day.

When a patient wakes up from an ECT treatment, he is usually confused for the first few minutes. Some patients may have a headache or some stiffness in their muscles, particularly after the first or second treatment, when the physician is still adjusting the amount of muscle relaxant needed. Most patients who receive ECT have some memory loss for the period when they were receiving the treatment. They may also have some difficulty remembering a few things that occurred just before the treatments began. These memory problems clear up completely after the ECT is stopped, however, and there is no evidence of any long-term effects on learning or memory.

In fact, ECT is probably the safest and most effective treatment available for depressive illness. It tends to be used only for hospitalized patients with relatively severe depression, however, since bad publicity has made both doctors and patients somewhat nervous about it. It is the treatment of choice for patients suffering concurrently from depression and heart disease, since tricyclics may activate adrenergic mechanisms in the heart in addition to those in the brain and therefore produce dangerous abnormalities in cardiac rhythm. It is much safer than tricyclics for depressed patients who have had recent heart attacks. Since it almost invariably produces rapid relief of depressive symptoms, some doctors also prefer to use it in patients who have made serious suicide attempts or are considered to be serious suicide risks.

The reluctance of both patients and doctors to accept the fact that ECT is a safe and effective treatment for depression is a sad commentary on the power of the media to influence our perceptions. It is also a sad commentary on the irrational responses that mental illness invokes in most people. It is hoped that the accurate information presented in this book, which attempts to describe fairly both the good and the bad effects of somatic therapies, will help to erase some of this misinformation and prejudice.

Treatment of Schizophrenia

The customary method of treating schizophrenia involves the use of antipsychotics or neuroleptics. Since the discovery of chlorpromazine, many other neuroleptics have been developed. Some of the more common ones include Thorazine, Mellaril, Stelazine, Navane, Prolixin, and Haldol. As in the case of the antidepressants, these drugs all appear to be about equally effective in relieving antipsychotic symptoms, and they differ primarily in their side effects. Mellaril and Thorazine are more sedating, Prolixin is more energizing, and Stelazine and Navane fall somewhere in the middle. As with the antidepressants, clinicians often try to use the side effects to advantage, prescribing the more sedating neuroleptics for agitated patients and the more energizing ones for withdrawn patients.

Dosages of neuroleptics vary widely since the drugs differ significantly in their "milligram potency" (the amount of antipsychotic effect included in a single milligram). Stelazine and Navane are about twenty times as potent as Thorazine, and Haldol is about fifty times as potent. The milligram potency has no real clinical significance, since doctors simply prescribe Thorazine in larger milligram doses, and no hazards are involved in taking these larger doses. The difference in milligram potency merely explains why one patient might be taking 800mg of an antipsychotic while another patient is taking only 10mg of a different antipsychotic.

The antipsychotics have many different types of side effects. Among the most troubling are the extrapyramidal or Parkinsonian side effects. As we have seen in chapter 5, both the basal ganglia and the limbic system are rich in dopaminergic neurons. Many neuroscientists believe that one major cause of schizophrenia is excessive dopamine transmission. The neuroleptics act by blocking dopamine transmission. We assume that the abnormality is in the limbic system and that the drugs exert their effect by decreasing dopamine transmission there. They do not block dopamine only in the limbic system, however; at the same time they cut down on dopamine transmission in the basal ganglia. The consequence is that patients receiving treatment with neuroleptics often have drug-induced symptoms like those of Parkinson's disease. Like patients suffering from Parkinson's disease, the patient receiving neuroleptics has a deficit of dopamine in his basal ganglia or extrapyramidal system.

The extrapyramidal symptoms are quite varied. One manifestation is a cluster of symptoms similar to those of Parkinson's disease, including tremor, rigidity, a masklike face, and a shuffling gait. Sometimes patients develop an unpleasant "dystonic reaction," which involves severe muscle spasms causing the head, fingers, toes, hands, arms, or legs, to twist to one side. Sometimes patients experience a great deal of physical restlessness, so that they cross and uncross their legs or move their arms and legs back and forth in stereotyped ways. Sometimes the restlessness is only internal, so that the patient *feels* agitated and may need to pace around, a symptom called "akathisia." Antipsychotics vary in the extent to which they produce these extrapyramidal side effects. In general, the side effects tend to be more severe with the more energizing drugs and less severe with the more sedating drugs. If these side effects become uncomfortable for the patient, they can be markedly decreased through the prescription of additional medications such as Cogentin that were developed originally to treat Parkinson's disease.

In addition to the extrapyramidal side effects, neuroleptics may have others that vary depending on the particular type of drug prescribed, such as sensitivity to the sun or the buildup of pigmentation in the skin. Patients who are taking neuroleptics and wish to learn more about these side effects should request information from their physicians.

One other infrequent, but relatively serious, side effect may occur as a result of taking neuroleptics, particularly when they have been taken for a long period of time. This side effect is called "tardive dyskinesia," an abnormal movement disorder that tends to persist sometimes even when the neuroleptics are discontinued (*tardive* = persistent; *dyskinesia* = abnormal movements). The most common form of these movements is a writhing or twisting of the muscles in the face and mouth. Similar writhing movements may occur in other parts of the body, however, such as the neck, arms, or hands. Sometimes these abnormal movements disappear when the medication is discontinued. If they do not, they may go away temporarily if the patient is placed on larger and larger doses of medication.

The cause of tardive dyskinesia is a matter of debate. One widely accepted theory, partially supported by research, suggests that neuroleptics induce an abnormal buildup of dopamine receptors in the basal ganglia, particularly the caudate, in an attempt to compensate for the dopamine blockade caused by neuroleptics. Tardive dyskinesia is not painful, but patients may feel it is embarrassing or disfiguring. Because of this potential long-term risk, many physicians and patients sometimes feel they are caught between Scylla and Charybdis. The neuroleptics are necessary in order to prevent recurrence or worsening of psychotic symptoms, which often reappear when the medication is discontinued. On the other hand, taking the medication may lead to this complication in a few patients. Most of the time, doctors and patients conclude that the benefit outweighs the risk. The risk may be diminished by reducing medication to the lowest dose necessary to control psychotic symptoms and by taking "drug holidays" under medical supervision from time to time.

When phenothiazines first appeared, doctors, patients, and their families all felt extraordinarily optimistic about the effect that these new drugs would have on the lives of people suffering from schizophrenia. It was widely believed that early aggressive treatment with antipsychotics would prevent further episodes or progressive deterioration. While this optimistic belief has proved true for some patients, it has not proved true for all. In some patients the disease appears to proceed inexorably—more slowly perhaps, but still inexorably. We now know that antipsychotics are not the wonder drugs that we once thought they were. They are very potent in decreasing hallucinations and often in cutting down on delusional thinking or even eliminating it, those types of symptoms sometimes referred to as "positive symptoms." Eileen Abbott, whose illness was described in chapter 4, is an example of a patient whose positive symptoms have been relatively well controlled by neuroleptics. On the other hand, negative or defect symptoms, such as alogia, affective flattening, or avolition, tend to be less responsive. Even the more energizing antipsychotics tend to have little effect on these negative symptoms. Roger Wallis, also described in chapter 4, is an example of a patient who has suffered from a negative type of schizophrenia that has responded less well to neuroleptics.

Treatment of the Anxiety Disorders

The schizophrenias and severe major affective disorders are usually treated with some form of somatic therapy. This is not always the case with the anxiety disorders, which may be treated with medication, behavioral therapy, psychotherapy, or a combination of two or three. Since the emphasis of this book is limited to biological approaches to psychiatry, this chapter discusses only the somatic therapy of anxiety disorders. This limitation, however, should not be taken to imply that other types of therapy are not appropriate as well.

The antianxiety drugs are among the most widely prescribed in medicine. The earliest was meprobamate or Miltown, but this medication has been largely supplanted by other, safer drugs such as Librium, Valium, Ativan, and Xanax. These drugs are widely used because they have specific calming or antianxiety effects without producing excessive sedation. People who take them find they feel less nervous and more relaxed, but without the side effects of other drugs that have been used in the past as relaxants. Alcohol, for example, is perhaps the world's oldest tranquilizer and antianxiety agent, but it produces intoxication in addition to relaxation, so that it affects thinking and motor activity. The barbiturates also produce relaxation, but they put people to sleep at the same time. The antianxiety drugs calm people without making them feel high, sleepy, or mentally and physically dulled.

The antianxiety drugs enjoy wide use because they have only minimal side effects and minimal long-term risks. Since they do not produce either a high or a great deal of sedation, they are not very popular drugs for abuse, unlike the barbiturates, narcotics, and amphetamines. They have a low toxicity, so there is little risk of accidental or intentional overdose, which is a high risk with barbiturates. In fact, the only serious long-term side effect observed with the antianxiety agents is psychological dependence and perhaps physiological dependence when taken in very high doses. Because of their powerful effects on anxiety, some people take these drugs over long periods of time and are reluctant to stop taking them because their anxiety is likely to recur on discontinuance. When the drugs are stopped abruptly after very large doses have been taken for a long time, patients sometimes show withdrawal symptoms such as tremulousness, agitation, or seizures.

The antianxiety drugs are used in psychiatry to relieve many different complaints and disorders. They are sometimes used to treat mild depression accompanied by anxiety; phobic disorder; panic disorder; post-traumatic stress disorder; and generalized anxiety disorder. These drugs clearly produce symptomatic relief, but there is considerable debate as to whether this symptomatic relief is desirable or whether it prevents people from understanding the psychological causes of their anxiety and learning to gain control over it by behavioral means. Some therapists have been concerned that these drugs may actually handicap the progress of therapy, since they provide the patient with a "crutch." Other therapists argue that patients often need a crutch in order to help wounds achieve their natural healing process; asking a patient to learn to gain control over a crippling phobia without some help in relieving anxiety is like asking a person with a broken leg to move around in a full cast without assistance from a crutch.

Evidence has accumulated that two other classes of drugs may be useful in treating some specific types of anxiety disorders, particularly panic disorder. These drugs are the tricyclics, particularly imipramine, and the MAOIs. Recent evidence suggests that Xanax may also have relatively specific effects on panic attacks. Consequently, many psychiatrists choose to prescribe these medications for patients who suffer from panic disorder, such as Greg Miller, whose case history was described in chapter 4.

Among the anxiety disorders, obsessive-compulsive disorder is perhaps the most difficult to treat. Some patients with obsessive-compulsive disorder respond relatively well to antianxiety drugs or to tricyclics. Some respond well to psychotherapy or behavioral therapy. Some clear up spontaneously, while a few, like Liz Antonelli of chapter 4, do not respond to anything and become steadily more crippled by their obsessions and compulsions as they grow older. Psychosurgery is sometimes used for patients who have suffered from incapacitating obsessions and compulsions for many years.

As noted in chapter 5, psychosurgery was developed by the Portuguese psychiatrist and neurologist Egas Moniz during the late 1930s and early 1940s. Although this surgical technique has usually been used relatively conservatively in Europe, it was adopted overenthusiastically in the United States during the 1950s for the treatment of agitated psychotic patients, particularly schizophrenics. In retrospect, the technique was used too frequently, and the surgical approach was relatively crude: Large amounts of frontal white-matter tracts were cut. Initially, it was noted that the patients indeed became calm, tranquil, and even uncaring; later it became obvious that they also had deficits in social judgment, creativity, and initiative.

As these facts emerged, the pendulum swung in the opposite direction in the United States, and people began to react to psychosurgery with revulsion. It continued to be used cautiously and infrequently for a few carefully selected cases in Great Britain and Europe. Likewise, a few centers in the United States also continued to use psychosurgery, primarily for the treatment of severe obsessive-compulsive disorder and occasionally for the treatment of intractable, incapacitating depression accompanied by anxiety.

Whereas the older technique of "prefrontal lobotomy" involved cutting large amounts of white-matter tracts, the modern technique of psychosurgery emphasizes the selective cutting of very tiny and quite specific portions of the tracts connecting the cingulate gyrus to the remainder of the limbic system. This technique is assumed to break up the reverberating circuits of the limbic system and thereby stop the self-perpetuating cycle of emotional stimulation that may be causing repetitive obsessions and compulsions. The cingulate gyrus was selected because it is the most accessible part of the limbic system. This procedure, called "cingulotomy," is not a panacea, but it is very helpful in some patients.

Immediately after cingulotomy, there are no obvious effects. However, as a few weeks pass, the patients gradually drop their obsessive-compulsive rituals, apparently without any discomfort; they simply no longer feel any need for them. Patients show no change in social judgment, personality, or creative or cognitive ability after cingulotomy. In fact, they tend to perform much better on standard psychological testing, such as IQ testing, because they are no longer handicapped by their obsessions and compulsions. For some reason, however, this technique does not help all obsessive-compulsive patients. The research done to date suggests that it is helpful in 50–60 percent of the cases treated. It should be emphasized that these are people who have had an extremely severe illness that has lasted for many years and has not responded to any treatment at all. After the surgery, these patients have been able to return to work and lead essentially normal lives.

Treatment of the Dementias

The affective disorders, schizophrenia, and anxiety disorders all have relatively well-established somatic therapies that are more or less successful. Unfortunately, there is as yet no well-established treatment for the dementias.

The underlying problem in dementia is an impairment in memory and other cognitive abilities, due to the loss of nerve cells in many different parts of the brain. Parkinson's disease, which is also characterized by the loss of nerve cells, has taught us that even when there is neuronal loss, the situation is not hopeless; drugs can be developed to supplement and assist transmission for the neurons that remain. Thus scientists hope that eventually a drug will be developed that will improve the memories and cognitive abilities of patients suffering from dementia. As we shall see in chapter 9, some evidence suggests that there is a particular loss in neurons that transmit by using acetylcholine. Clinicians have experimented with giving demented patients choline in a manner analogous to giving L-dopa to the Parkinsonian patient. This appears to help minimally in a few cases, but it is clear that choline does not provide the same degree of help for dementia that L-dopa provides for the person suffering from Parkinson's disease. Thus the search for new antidementia drugs continues.

In the meantime, psychiatrists are limited to using medications that may help in controlling some of the associated symptoms of dementia. While the underlying abnormality is a deficit in memory and cognition, patients suffering from dementia are also frequently irritable, agitated, suspicious, and depressed. These associated symptoms are sometimes relieved by antipsychotics or antidepressants. Usually these medications must be given in somewhat smaller doses to elderly patients than would be used for younger, healthier people. A person with an early mild dementia accompanied by depression may feel better for several years if treated with low doses of tricyclics. A mildly demented patient who is suspicious and irritable, thereby causing considerable pain and grief to her spouse or other family members, may improve on low doses of antipsychotics and be cared for within her own home for many years. Haldol has been found to be particularly useful in minimizing the behavioral problems associated with dementia, since it is less likely to lower blood pressure than some of the other drugs. (A drop in blood pressure, reducing nourishment to the brain, is the last thing that a person trying to function on a reduced number of neurons needs.)

A final word should be said about the fact that some cases of dementia *are* reversible. Until we have genuine antidementia drugs available, the classical dementias, such as Alzheimer's disease or Huntington's chorea, will fall into the category of irreversible illnesses whose inexorable course cannot be halted. On the other hand, some illnesses tend to mimic these classical dementias and yet are due to other causes. Sometimes a severe depression looks very much like a classical dementia, since a person who is quite depressed can have poor concentration, be inattentive, and appear to have poor memory. If an astute clinician recognizes the possibility of the depressive syndrome from such clues as a rather abrupt onset or a family history of affective disorder, she may place the patient on antidepressants and apparently produce a miraculous cure for a dementia. In fact, she has cured a well-recognized phenomenon known as "depressive pseudodementia." Other medical diseases, such as hypothyroidism, may also closely resemble the classical dementias. Before giving up and assuming that the patient has a classical dementia, everyone involved should feel sure that a treatable and reversible dementia has been ruled out.

9

THE REVOLUTION IN RESEARCH:

The Search for Causes

> More needs she the divine than the physician.
> God, god forgive us all!
>
> WILLIAM SHAKESPEARE,
> —Comment of the physician called
> to treat Lady Macbeth's madness
> in *Macbeth*

What causes mental illness?

Only a few centuries ago, the answer to that question was easy: The mentally ill were sinners in the hands of an angry God, souls in torment who had sold themselves to Satan, people who through their own free will had been careless with their lives and their bodies. At best they were led too easily into temptation, and at worst they had willfully chosen to follow the evil forces now controlling them. Their muttering conversations with the voices they heard, their immobilized misery, their descriptions of persecutory torment were all taken as evidence of the presence of diabolical forces, making them objects of fear and derision. A few people, like Lady Macbeth's physician, looked upon the mentally ill with pity as well. But nearly everyone assumed that mental illness was a "spiritual disease," that it was caused by supernatural rather than natural forces, and that its victims were somehow responsible for their own suffering.

Although these attitudes are changing, they continue to linger. Unlike almost every other type of illness, mental illnesses still tend to carry an aura of guilt and moral responsibility. Even today many people suspect that a person who is mentally ill must have brought his problems on himself and that he could cure himself if he would just "shape up." Parents of teen-agers suffering from schizophrenia or depression wonder what they have done wrong, blaming themselves for being too strict and inducing excessive guilt in their child—or too permissive and not instilling enough self-control. A person who misses work for treatment of cancer is accorded sympathy and pity, but a person who is hospitalized for mental illness may return to find his job lost, his license to practice law or medicine temporarily revoked, or his place in graduate school gone. Even people who pay lip service to enlightened attitudes toward mental illness may find that its actual presence in their lives evokes feelings of fear or inchoate glimmerings of moral indignation. The person who is mentally ill must carry a double burden: He must experience the actual suffering of the illness and he must sometimes experience the punishments for being ill that society still feels he must deserve.

These attitudes persist because people remain confused about the nature and causes of mental illness. Frightening diseases have always caused revulsion or reproach. In biblical times the victim of leprosy —a disease that produces ugly deformities, especially of the face—was treated as a social outcast, and his illness was thought to be due to demonic possession. In the nineteenth century, people realized that leprosy was due to infection with the leprosy bacillus; leper colonies continued to exist because the disease was contagious, but the social isolation was no longer seen as a form of punishment. Still, leprosy was more feared than another, more common disease, tuberculosis, caused by a similar type of germ but producing no obvious physical deformity. Unlike its cousin, leprosy, tuberculosis (or "consumption") was even a rather glamorous way to die, memorialized in the poetry of Keats and the music of *La Bohème.* Leprosy, because it produces deformity and makes people appear inhuman, has remained one of the most dreaded of diseases, although it is now clearly seen as an illness rather than a consequence of sin.

Like leprosy, mental illness strikes at something that is specifically and peculiarly human. Leprosy rots away the face and hands. Mental illness affects the personality, the way people relate to one another, and the way they think and talk. It *does* seem to affect the spirit, the psyche, the soul. Confusion about the causes of mental illness has arisen because many people tend to assume there must be a dichotomy between the mind and the body, and that a disease of the mind must be different from a disease of the body. People cannot help what happens to their bodies, but they *can* control their minds or spirits.

As the foregoing chapters of this book have shown, the mind and body are in fact inseparable. The word *mind* refers to those functions of the body that reside in the brain. When we talk, think, feel, or dream, each of these mental functions is due to electrical impulses passing through the complicated and highly specialized electrical circuits that make up the human brain. The messages passed along these circuits are transmitted and modulated primarily through chemical processes. Mental illnesses are due to disruptions in the normal flow of messages through this circuitry, and these "breaks" in the brain can occur in many different ways. The nerves forming command centers may become ill or wear out and die. The wires may lose their insulation. Some neurons may in a sense become "overheated" and send or receive too many chemical messages. Short circuits may occur so that new connections are formed that should not be there, or command centers may become disconnected from one another through the loss of the wiring between them. To make matters still more complicated, this electrical circuitry exists in a living organism, and so it is adaptable and dynamic. When a break occurs in a system, the body and its brain often possess the capacity to heal themselves in various compensatory ways, such as developing new circuits to replace broken connections, sending in inhibitory chemicals to cool down overheated circuits, or growing more receptors to enhance transmission when it seems to be slowing down. Mental illness is truly a nervous breakdown—a breakdown that occurs when the nerves of the brain have an injury so severe that their own internal healing capacities cannot repair it.

While the illnesses that these "breaks" in the brain produce may affect capacities that are peculiarly and intensely human, they are breaks in the biology of the body, breaks that have usually passed beyond a person's capacity to heal himself. This fact produces a startling shift in our perceptions of moral responsibility for mental illness. The victim of mental illness has not brought it on himself, and he cannot cure it through his own free will. To ask the victim of schizophrenia to "shape up" or exert more self-control is about as fair (and medically sound) as asking a person who has recently suffered a heart attack to try to run up another flight of stairs.

What Is a Cause?

Figuring out what causes illnesses is not as simple as it might seem. For example, what "causes" pneumonia? The easy answer is infection with the *pneumococcus,* a germ that frequently produces pneumonia. When a patient is suffering from the symptoms of pneumonia, it can be proved that it is caused by the *pneumococcus* if that germ is found to be present in large quantities when the patient's sputum is cultured in the laboratory. If many germs of this type are present, the patient is said to have pneumococcal pneumonia, a disease caused by infection with the pneumococcal bacillus.

But if this germ causes pneumonia, why doesn't the doctor caring for the patient catch pneumonia from her? Germs of many kinds are all around us, and yet very few of us get sick from them. Germs may cause disease, but only if they fall on fallow ground. There are various predisposing factors that make it more likely for someone to develop pneumonia. For example, people are more susceptible to the *pneumococcus* if they are older, if their immune reactions are reduced through some other illness or through taking medications such as steroids, or if their lungs have been damaged through smoking cigarettes. Thus many different factors must be present in order to cause pneumonia, and therefore the causes are said to be "multifactorial." (Like journalists, advertising agents, and sports commentators, doctors also have their favorite clichés. One of these is the word *multifactorial.* It covers an extraordinary expanse of ignorance.)

Most diseases *are* probably caused by multiple factors, some of them physical, some of them environmental, and some of them hereditary. Disentangling these various kinds of causes from one another can be a difficult scientific problem. For example, people who suffer from heart attacks are more likely to have been smokers, to have eaten a diet rich in cholesterol or salt, to exercise infrequently and pursue sedentary occupations, and to have parents who also suffer from cardiovascular disease. Each of these factors is in some sense a cause, and yet none alone is a cause; some peculiar and shifting combination of them is required to produce disease. Even the issue of moral responsibility may enter in. In a sense, a person who smokes cigarettes and knows that smoking increases the risk of heart disease can be said to have helped to cause a heart attack through her own free choice. (Yet whatever people may say about mental illness, they never accuse heart-attack victims of causing their own illnesses.) In any case, when one looks closely at the causes of illness, they can spread out to a very wide range indeed.

One may also note that the causes of disease can penetrate to many different levels. One can recite glibly that pneumonia is caused by the *pneumococcus,* adding the more sophisticated qualifications that an overwhelming number of these germs must invade a particularly vulnerable host for disease to occur, and that other types of germs besides the *pneumococcus* may also infect the lungs and cause pneumonia. But in another sense, one might explain the causes of disease in terms of what these germs actually do to the body and its cells. One might describe how germs enter cells in the lungs, produce inflammation and an excessive production of fluids, and thereby prevent the exchange of carbon dioxide and oxygen. The germs cause the cells that breathe for us to drown in their own juices. In one sense, one can say the pneumonia has been caused by the presence of a germ. In another sense, one can say it is caused by the way the presence of the germ causes the normal functioning of the cells in the lungs to break down. One can explain causes in terms of whether or not they are present, and one can explain them in terms of how they actually work to produce damage. Although the second type of explanation is the subtler and more interesting one, we do not always understand it well for many serious medical diseases, such as cancer.

The causes of mental illness are clearly multifactorial and, like cancer, are at present only partially understood. The story told in this chapter is a bit like one in a difficult modern novel. We know pieces of the plot and have many conflicting ideas about the cast of characters involved. The general shape of the story is clear: The various forms of mental illness are due to many different types of brain abnormalities, including the loss of nerve cells and excesses and deficits in chemical transmission between neurons; sometimes the fault may be in the pattern of the wiring or circuitry, sometimes in the command centers, and sometimes in the way messages move along the wires. The tendency to develop these abnormalities may run in families and therefore be partially hereditary, but it is also clearly due to a broad range of environmental factors, which may include infection with viruses, abnormalities in the nourishment the brain receives, head injuries, or even the shocks and stresses of everyday life. It is caused by a wide variety of "breaks" in the brain. The psychological or social terms used to describe these breaks, such as *loss of ego boundaries* or *lack of self-esteem,* are metaphors used to describe biological processes that we are just beginning to understand.

What Causes Schizophrenia?

Since schizophrenia is a crippling disease that usually begins relatively early in life and maims without killing, the search for its causes is perhaps the highest priority in modern psychiatry. Schizophrenia probably produces more hours and years of suffering than any disease that human beings must bear. If we understand its causes, we will be able to find better treatments, and perhaps even ways to prevent it.

The current evidence concerning the causes of schizophrenia is a mosaic. It is quite clear that multiple factors are involved. These include changes in the chemistry of the brain, changes in the structure of the brain, and genetic factors. Viral infections and head injuries may also play a role. Some of these may be predisposing factors rather than actual causes. Some may be actual causes but will not produce disease unless helped along by predisposing factors; this type of cause is often called "necessary but not sufficient." (In the instance of pneumonia, the *pneumococcus* is an example of this type of cause.) Some may be causes in the sense that they represent observed changes in the brain, while others may be causes in the sense that they represent the underlying mechanisms producing the illness at the cellular level. Finally, schizophrenia is probably a heterogeneous group of diseases, some of which are caused by one factor and some by another.

NEUROCHEMICAL FACTORS

Changes in the chemistry of the brain are almost certainly present in some types of schizophrenia. The most widely accepted theory concerning the neurochemical abnormalities involved is called "the dopamine hypothesis." According to this hypothesis, schizophrenia is due to overactive transmission in the circuitry of the brain that uses dopamine as its chemical messenger. As we saw in chapter 5, dopamine is an important chemical messenger in many parts of the limbic system, the portion of the brain that governs aspects of emotion and personality that are thought to go awry in schizophrenia. The dopamine hypothesis, like all our current theories concerning the causes of mental illness, is just that—a hypothesis. That is, it has what scientists refer to as "heuristic value" in that it explains many observations about the nature of schizophrenia and is useful in generating research into its causes. It has received strong support from many different types of research studies, but it is not as yet *proved* so that it has become a fact rather than a hypothesis.

The first suggestion that dopamine transmission might be abnormal in schizophrenia came through the development of the antipsychotic drugs. It was clear that these drugs significantly reduced the symptoms of schizophrenia. How did they work? Early investigators noticed that animals treated with neuroleptics tended to produce an outpouring of dopamine. At a naïve level, one might conclude that the drugs worked by increasing the amount of dopamine transmission in the brain and that schizophrenia (like Parkinson's disease) is due to insufficient dopamine. Nothing is quite this simple, however, as several clever early investigators realized. Instead, they suspected that this outpouring of dopamine occurred in response to blockade of the dopamine receptor. The new neuroleptic drugs would literally move in and sit on the receptor sites of neurons destined to receive messages, thereby preventing them from accepting any that were being sent through the neurotransmitter dopamine. The transmitter neurons, realizing that their messages were not being received, responded by sending out even more dopamine, but these massive amounts of dopamine could still not get through because the receptors were still blocked.

When this theory was developed during the 1960s, the dopamine receptor was just a gleam in the neuroscientist's eye. It had to be there, but no one had been able to see it, because the technology was not available. A few years later, however, special laboratory techniques were developed so that specific chemicals could be used to find receptor sites for dopamine in nerve cells. These techniques could then be used to map the location of dopamine-receptor sites in the brain, to determine whether or not the receptor sites were blocked, and to determine whether the number of dopamine receptors had increased or decreased either in patients suffering from schizophrenia or in response to treatment with drugs. As the story has spun itself out during recent years, it has emerged that there are even several different kinds of dopamine receptors, only one of which (called the "D2 receptor") appears to transmit messages producing schizophrenic symptoms, is blocked by neuroleptics effective in treating schizophrenia, and is present in increased numbers in patients suffering from schizophrenia.

The early version of the dopamine hypothesis suggested that patients suffering from schizophrenia had excessive dopaminergic transmission in the limbic system. This excessive transmission could be due to several different things. One possibility was the excessive production of dopamine by messenger neurons. Another was excessive sensitivity to dopamine by the neurons programmed to receive messages. A third possibility was that dopamine was produced in normal amounts and that the receptor neurons were normal, but that something had broken down in the processes used to destroy dopamine after it had served its function of transmitting messages.

Most of the early research exploring these three variations of the dopamine hypothesis involved determining where dopamine transmission was occurring in the brain and the degree to which it was blocked by neuroleptics in animals. Obviously, one must make a large inferential leap in order to generalize about mental illness in humans based on research using the brains of rats. More recently, however, our knowledge of neurochemical "breaks" in schizophrenia has been strengthened through the study of actual human brains. In several centers throughout the world, investigators have amassed large "brain banks"—collections of brains from people known to have had specific types of mental illness who have granted permission for their brains to be studied scientifically after their death. Since it is difficult to generalize from animals to man, and since it is ethically forbidden to do most types of experimentation on the human brain while people are still alive, these brain banks provide a rich resource for the study of mechanisms in mental illness. The brains collected in these scientific banks are referred to as "postmortem brains" (brains after death).

The combination of research on the effects of drugs in animals, the effects in human beings, and the study of postmortem brains has led to further refinements in the dopamine hypothesis. The animal research has been used to explore which neuroleptics are most powerful in blocking dopamine receptors. The drugs that produce the strongest blockade in animals are also those that are most effective in reducing the symptoms of schizophrenia in human beings. Further, several drugs that are powerful dopamine antagonists, such as reserpine, may also significantly reduce the symptoms of schizophrenia, although they are rarely used clinically because of side effects or other reasons. On the other hand, drugs known to enhance dopamine transmission, such as amphetamines, are likely to cause or exacerbate the symptoms of schizophrenia. All these pieces of research support the likelihood that the dopamine system has broken down in schizophrenia.

The postmortem research has, however, given the strongest support to the dopamine hypothesis and also pointed more specifically to the nature of the abnormality. When scientists have examined the brains of schizophrenic patients after death, the primary abnormality they have found is an increased number of dopamine receptors in the basal ganglia and the limbic system. These results suggest that schizophrenics have "overheated circuits" in their limbic systems because the neurons programmed to receive messages have a larger number of receptors and therefore are oversensitive. As soon as this exciting discovery was noted, a concern was raised that the increase in dopamine receptors might be due to treatment with neuroleptics rather than an abnormality causing schizophrenia. Although the matter is by no means settled, an increased number of dopamine receptors has been found in postmortem brains of schizophrenic patients who were never treated with any type of medication, providing support for the possibility that at least some patients suffering from schizophrenia develop symptoms because of excessive dopamine transmission and specifically because of excessive numbers of dopamine receptors.

STRUCTURAL ABNORMALITIES

Patients suffering from schizophrenia have also been noted to have brain abnormalities at the larger structural level. As chapter 7 has described, clinicians and investigators have begun to study the brains of patients suffering from schizophrenia using the new brain-imaging techniques that have become available during the past ten years. During future years, some of these techniques will no doubt be used to map neurochemical abnormalities with the PET scanner, but as yet the resolution of the PET scanner is not high enough nor the neurochemical techniques advanced enough to permit studies of living brains at this relatively fine cellular level. To date, these techniques have been used to explore larger structural changes.

As chapter 7 has indicated, research using brain-imaging techniques suggests that some patients suffering from schizophrenia have visible structural abnormalities that can be seen using CT scanning. The abnormality noted most consistently is enlargement of the ventricles. This ventricular enlargement is presumably due to shrinkage of the brain because neurons have died; the fluid-filled ventricles have grown to fill the empty space as the brain has shrunk. Less commonly, the cortical sulci are also enlarged, another indication of shrinkage or atrophy. Enlargement of the ventricles suggests that the atrophy may be in deep subcortical gray matter such as the thalamus, parts of the limbic system, or the basal ganglia. Sulcal enlargement suggests that the cortex has also atrophied. The finding that schizophrenic patients have structural brain changes has been reported repeatedly by investigators throughout the world during the past ten years. The frequency of structural abnormalities varies from study to study, however, depending on how the abnormality is defined and the type of patient studied. The rate of ventricular enlargement reported in patients suffering from schizophrenia ranges from 10 to 50 percent.

In general, the structural abnormalities appear to be present in those patients who are more chronically ill and who have more social and intellectual deterioration. However, the abnormalities have also been found in young schizophrenic patients when they were being seen for the first time and had not yet received any type of treatment. Patients with ventricular enlargement tend to show some indication of poor adjustment even during early childhood, such as lack of interest in making friends or participating in school activities. Patients with ventricular enlargement may also be less likely to respond to neuroleptic medication.

As chapter 7 has indicated, brain-imaging techniques can also be used to search for other types of structural abnormalities—for example, abnormal enlargement of crucial brain structures such as the limbic system or the corpus callosum. These small structures could not be seen clearly on the older CT-scanning equipment, and insufficient numbers of patients have been studied as yet with the new high-resolution CT scanners or with NMR in order to determine whether other types of structural abnormalities can be seen in the "living brain" as well.

GENETIC FACTORS

People have recognized for centuries that mental illness sometimes runs in families. That observation suggests that the tendency to develop mental illness may be inherited—or, in the language of science, it may be caused by genetic transmission. The genetic information that makes all of us the particular individuals that we are is programmed on forty-six chromosomes that are present in the nucleus of each cell in our bodies. We have received half these chromosomes from our mothers and half from our fathers. Many aspects of our lives are under a high degree of genetic control, such as our hair and eye color, our height and weight, and perhaps even our personalities and abilities.

But for many important aspects of our lives, these genetic factors interact with other nongenetic factors so that it is often difficult to disentangle heredity from environment, or nature from nurture. For example, each of us was probably born with a genetic program that dictated the height to which we would grow—more or less. This program could be modulated, however, by a whole range of environmental factors. For example, eating a splendidly nourishing diet throughout childhood and early adulthood might add a few extra inches, whereas exposure to environmental poisons or repeated infections during childhood might lop off an inch or two. For a trait such as height, the genetic commands tend to set the zenith and the low point, while environmental influences help determine where we actually fall within this range.

A few aspects of our lives are under an extremely high degree of genetic determination, such as the color of our eyes or the tendency to develop a few very rare diseases. Most aspects of our lives, however, including the tendency to develop mental illnesses and most other diseases, are probably more like height and weight: They are due to a mixture of nature and nurture.

As far as we know at this point, most forms of schizophrenia are to some extent hereditary, but only to a mild degree. The earliest investigations of genetic factors in schizophrenia involved the use of a technique known as the "family study." In family studies, a person with a particular type of illness is identified, and then other members of his family are also evaluated in order to determine whether or not they have had the same illness. If many members of the family tend to suffer from the illness, then it is highly familial and possibly hereditary or genetic. Early studies of the relatives of schizophrenic patients indicated that about 5 percent of their parents had schizophrenia and about 10 percent of their brothers and sisters or their children were ill. The disorder occurs in only about 1 percent of the general population, so the rate of schizophrenia is clearly higher in the families of schizophrenic patients.

But is this due to nature or nurture or both? A higher rate of illness in the relatives of schizophrenics could be due to environmental rather than genetic causes. Did some people develop schizophrenia from the strain of living with a schizophrenic relative? Did some relatives develop the illness through the influence of role modeling or by gradually learning and accepting psychotic beliefs? After the early family studies suggested a possible familial factor in schizophrenia, investigators began to use other, more sophisticated methods for examining whether it was caused by genes or by environmental factors.

One such method is the study of twins. Since identical twins share exactly the same genetic material, they should be identical (or nearly so) in any aspect of their lives that is genetically determined, particularly if they are reared in more or less the same environment. The rate of agreement between a pair of twins in their tendency to develop a particular characteristic, such as an illness like schizophrenia, is called the "concordance rate." If 150 pairs of twins are studied and they all are identical for a certain trait, then the concordance rate is said to be 100 percent. If 75 pairs of twins are identical for the trait and 75 are not (i.e., are discordant), then the concordance rate is only 50 percent. Twins provide an interesting "laboratory" for studying the genetics of mental illness, because identical or monozygotic (MZ) twins can be compared with nonidentical or dizygotic (DZ) twins in order to determine the degree to which a particular trait is hereditary. While monozygotic twins have identical genes, only 50 percent of the genes are identical in dizygotic twins. One can compare the concordance rates in monozygotic and dizygotic twins to get an indication of the degree to which a trait is genetically determined. For disorders that are totally genetic, the concordance rate in MZ twins should be 100 percent and the rate in DZ twins 50 percent. If the rate is lower, then one knows that the disorder is not totally controlled by genetic factors.

Twin studies of schizophrenia have yielded some very interesting findings. When one member of a pair of identical twins develops schizophrenia, the odds that the other twin will develop it are about 50 percent. If schizophrenia were totally genetic, the odds should be 100 percent. The fact that the concordance rate for schizophrenia among identical twins is only 50 percent indicates that the tendency to develop schizophrenia is only partly determined by genetic factors. If one then examines nonidentical twins, one finds that the concordance rate drops to 10 or 15 percent, about the same that one would find among siblings. This makes sense, since nonidentical twins are basically siblings who were born at the same time.

While the study of identical and nonidentical twins has told us a great deal about the extent to which schizophrenia is hereditary, it has not told the whole story. Scientists were quick to point out that studying twins did not give a pure separation of nature and nurture, since twins generally grow up in the same environment and might even model themselves after one another because of the psychological effect of being a twin. Consequently, within the past few years an imaginative new research design was introduced that separated heredity and environment more clearly. This method involved studying children born to schizophrenic mothers but adopted and reared by normal families. In order to control for the possible psychological effects of being adopted, these adopted children of schizophrenics were compared with children born to normal mothers and adopted and reared by adoptive parents who had no evidence of mental illness.

In these studies, the effects of environment were held completely constant. These two samples—the children of schizophrenic mothers and the children of normal mothers—provided a laboratory in which the role of heredity could be studied completely separately from the role of environment. If schizophrenia were hereditary, rather than due to learning or role modeling, then one would expect a higher rate of schizophrenic illness in the children of the schizophrenic mothers than in the children of the normal mothers. If schizophrenia were caused wholly by genetic influences (which the twin studies have already told us is not the case), then 50 percent of the adopted children of schizophrenic mothers would develop schizophrenia, while only 1 percent (the general population rate) of the children of normal mothers would do so. In fact, the rate turned out to be about 10:1. As in the case of the twin studies, this rate is high enough to again indicate that genetic factors are important, but not high enough to indicate that they control the whole story.

One is bound to conclude from these various studies of the genetics of schizophrenia that hereditary factors play a role, but they are not all-important. What, then, are the other factors thought likely to produce schizophrenia? One hypothesis that has been proposed is that schizophrenia may be due to a viral illness occurring early in life and producing some type of mild encephalitis, or brain inflammation, that predisposes to the development of schizophrenia. This hypothesis has been supported in part by studies of viruslike agents in the cerebrospinal fluid of schizophrenics. It has also been supported by the fact that schizophrenia is more common among people born during the winter months, when viral illnesses occur with a particular frequency. Another factor that might predispose to the development of schizophrenia is a difficult labor and delivery, which could produce mild brain damage. A modest amount of evidence also suggests that patients suffering from schizophrenia may be somewhat more likely to have mild or "soft" signs of head injury or brain damage occurring early in life.

The causes of schizophrenia are like a difficult and only partially solved puzzle. We know that schizophrenics may have chemical imbalances in their brains—in particular, excessive transmission in the dopamine system. Some patients also have structural changes, as evidenced by ventricular enlargement. The neurochemical abnormalities can be corrected, at least partially, through treatment with neuroleptics, but there is no way to rebuild a brain that has suffered structural damage, and in fact patients with signs of structural damage tend to respond poorly to the chemical treatments currently available.

These bits of evidence suggest that there may be at least two different types of schizophrenia, and possibly more. One type, sometimes referred to as "florid" or "positive" schizophrenia, is characterized by prominent "positive" symptoms, such as delusions and hallucinations, that tend to respond relatively well to neuroleptic treatment. These patients may suffer from "neurochemical" schizophrenia, or schizophrenia confined to the limbic system. Another type of schizophrenia, characterized by prominent "negative" or defect symptoms, such as blunted affect and impoverished speech, may be due to diffuse structural damage to the brain, as manifested by ventricular enlargement on CT scanning. Both types of schizophrenia involve "breaks" in the brain, but the breaks are quite different from one another in their nature and implications. Genetics, viral infections, and head injury could be predisposing or contributing factors for either of these two types of schizophrenia, with some being more prominent in one subtype than in another.

What Causes Affective Disorders?

Chapter 4 described two major subtypes of affective disorder: mania and depression. Since depression is such a common illness, affecting between 10 and 25 percent of the population, it has received much more attention from researchers than has mania, which affects .5 to 1 percent of the population. The story of the search for the causes of depression runs parallel to that just described for schizophrenia in many respects.

NEUROCHEMICAL FACTORS

While people suspected for many years that some type of chemical imbalance might be causing the symptoms of depression, it was only after the modern era of psychopharmacology began, in the 1950s and 1960s, that this theory could be explored scientifically. As soon as drugs appeared that had obvious effects on the brain and on the symptoms of mental illness, scientists could begin to examine how these drugs actually worked, hoping that this research would eventually be used to eliminate the underlying causes of the illness.

This research with drugs led to the formulation of the "catecholamine hypothesis" about the cause of affective disorder. Like the dopamine hypothesis, the catecholamine hypothesis is theory rather than fact, although it too enjoys substantial scientific support. The catecholamine hypothesis, in its simplest early form, stated that depression was due to a deficiency of norepinephrine, one of the major catecholamine systems in the brain described in chapter 5, while mania might be due to an excess of norepinephrine.

Unlike dopamine, which occurs primarily in the brain, the catecholamines are very active in the peripheral nervous system—the part of the nervous system outside the brain that governs bodily activities such as heart rate and blood pressure. The part of the peripheral nervous system that uses these neurotransmitters is also sometimes called the "sympathetic nervous system," its primary activity being to produce arousal and alertness and to generally speed things up. It is the sympathetic nervous system that swings into action when we are threatened in some way, and so it is said to prepare the body for "fight or flight." The sympathetic nerves increase heart rate, strengthen the pumping action of the heart, and dilate the pupils of the eyes so that we can see better. The effects of the sympathetic nervous system are countered by those of the parasympathetic system, which generally slows things down. In a sense, the effects of catecholamines in the peripheral nervous system provide a hint as to how they might work in the brain.

The catecholamine theory received some support as the mechanisms of the new antidepressant drugs were illuminated. Both types of drugs used to treat depression—the tricyclics and the monoamine-oxidase inhibitors—tend to increase the amount of norepinephrine available in the central nervous system, although they work in somewhat different ways.

Their mechanism of action is illustrated in figure 29. This figure portrays a transmitter neuron attempting to send messages across a synapse to a receptor neuron using the norepinephrine. Norepinephrine is stored in tiny sacs, which are called "synaptic vesicles," inside the messenger neurons. When the neuron receives a command to fire and release norepinephrine, the synaptic vesicles open and send norepinephrine out into the synapse. This norepinephrine travels to the receptor sites on the receptor neuron, thereby sending its message on.

Naturally, some norepinephrine remains in the area of the synapse. In order to prevent waste and maintain sufficient stores of norepinephrine inside the messenger neurons, some of it travels back to the messenger neuron and reenters synaptic vesicles. Some is also metabolized (or broken down chemically and therefore made ineffec-

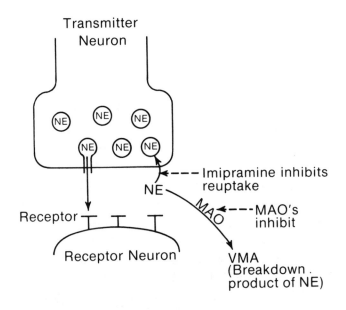

Fig. 29. Schematic representation of actions of antidepressant drugs.

tive) into 3-methoxy, 4-hydroxymandelic acid (vanilmandelicacid, VMA) through a chemical enzyme circulating in the synapse, known as monoamine oxidase (MAO). Both the tricyclics and monoamine-oxidase inhibitors (MAOIs) work by increasing the amount of norepinephrine available in the norepinephrine transmitter system. The MAOIs block the action of monoamine oxidase, thereby preventing norepinephrine from being destroyed and increasing the amount available for transmission. The tricyclics work by preventing the norepinephrine present in the synaptic cleft from being returned to the transmitter neuron and its synaptic vesicles, thereby increasing the amount of norepinephrine continually available in the synapse and thus enhancing transmission and excitation.

This research on the mechanism of drug actions has been done primarily in animals. Again, we need to know about norepinephrine in human beings, and in particular human beings suffering from depression, before we can be sure that animal research can really tell us anything about the mechanisms of mental illness. One approach has involved studying one of the breakdown products of norepinephrine, MHPG, which comes primarily from the brain. (MHPG has already been mentioned in chapter 7.) One can measure the amount of

MHPG in the urine and get a rough indication of whether or not norepinephrine is decreased in the brains of patients suffering from depression. When urinary MHPG was examined, it was found that some depressed patients, particularly those with severe melancholic depression or bipolar patients in the depressed phase, tended to have lower MHPG. Thus the catecholamine hypothesis has received some support from research in human beings with mental illness. It should be noted, however, that not all patients with depression have low MHPG.

The catecholamine hypothesis has been supplemented by another hypothesis, the "serotonin hypothesis." Serotonin is also a major transmitter in the central nervous system. Unlike dopamine, which is well localized to specific areas, serotonin and norepinephrine tend to throw up a wide net with endings scattered in many parts of the brain, as figures 15, 16, and 17 have illustrated in chapter 5. This pattern of distribution suggests that both these transmitter systems may have a general modulating effect, probably working to excite or alert. Like norepinephrine, serotonin transmission is also stimulated by antidepressant drugs. The tricyclics increase the amount of serotonin available at the synapse by preventing reuptake, just as they do for norepinephrine. The principal breakdown product of serotonin is 5-hydroxyindoleacetic acid (5-HIAA). Urinary 5-HIAA is a poor index of brain serotonin activity, but its presence in the spinal fluid can be used to explore the possibility of a serotonin deficit in depression. This has been done by collecting samples of CSF from depressed patients through a "spinal tap," a relatively simple technique for examining human CSF. Much as in the case of norepinephrine, a subgroup of depressed patients (approximately 45 percent) have been found to have low 5-HIAA.

These two hypotheses combine to suggest the possibility that there may be two subtypes of depressive illness: one due to norepinephrine deficiency and the other to a serotonin deficiency in the brain. This possibility is supported by the fact that some antidepressants, such as desipramine, work principally by enhancing norepinephrine transmission; while others, such as chlomipramine, seem to enhance serotonin transmission.

The catecholamine theory of depression was once supplemented by a corollary hypothesis suggesting that manic patients had excessive norepinephrine transmission occurring in their brains. This corollary, however, has received very little research support. Manic patients do not produce increased amounts of catecholamine metabolites in their urine or cerebrospinal fluid.

NEUROENDOCRINE ABNORMALITIES

As chapter 7 has already described, during recent years investigators have also noted that depressed patients appear to have another, possibly related type of chemical imbalance in their brains. This imbalance involves the regulation of endocrine function through secretions that arise in the hypothalamic part of the brain and pass on to the pituitary gland, the little saclike structure buried deep inside the head. The pituitary sends out hormones, or chemical messengers, that are circulated through the blood to target organs such as the thyroid, the adrenal glands, and the ovaries. It also controls several other endocrine systems, such as growth hormone (which regulates bodily growth and the level of sugar in the blood), melanin secretion (which governs skin pigmentation), and prolactin (which in women stimulates milk secretion from the breasts and contraction of the uterus).

Chapter 7 described in detail the abnormalities in cortisol secretion that have been observed in patients suffering from depression. A substantial number of depressed patients produce large amounts of cortisol, and they are unable to cut down on this excessive cortisol production when given dexamethasone, a drug that suppresses cortisol secretion in normal people. The excessive secretion of cortisol and the inability to suppress normally point to some kind of defect in the pituitary, the hypothalamus, or still higher centers that regulate the hypothalamus.

The abnormalities in cortisol secretion do not exist in isolation, however. Investigators have also observed other types of failure in neuroendocrine modulation and secretion. In addition to the dexamethasone-suppression test, other types of "challenge" tests have been given experimentally. For example, normal people given insulin will have a drop in their blood sugar. When this occurs, growth-hormone secretion is increased and blood sugar is raised back up again to normal levels. When depressed patients are given this "insulin tolerance test," however, some are unable to produce a normal outpouring of growth hormone. Another type of challenge test involves giving thyrotropin-releasing hormone (TRH). Normal people respond to this stimulus by producing increased amounts of thyroid-stimulating hormone (TSH), but some depressed patients do not. Depressed patients may show a similar blunting of response when given challenge tests to produce more prolactin. Thus they appear to be defective in many types of neuroendocrine secretion.

What do all these neuroendocrine abnormalities mean? As usual, the answers are not yet fully known, and they are not likely to be simple. The pattern of abnormality suggests that the defects do not lie in target organs, such as the adrenals or thyroid, or even in the pituitary gland itself. Rather, they are probably at the level of the hypothalamus, the command center governing the pituitary, or at some even higher level. Messages sent from other parts of the brain to the hypothalamus usually use the norepinephrine system. Likewise, dopamine and norepinephrine are the neurotransmitters used by the hypothalamus to talk to the pituitary. It is therefore possible that all the neuroendocrine abnormalities in depression could be explained through the catecholamine hypothesis—that is, depressed patients have a defect in norepinephrine transmission that impairs their ability to regulate the secretion of all types of hormones. While this explanation is simple, parsimonious, and consistent with other theories about the causes of depression, it may turn out to be an oversimplification.

GENETIC FACTORS

The same types of increasingly sophisticated methods used to study genetic factors in schizophrenia have also been employed to examine the nature-versus-nurture controversy in the affective disorders. The results indicate that, if anything, affective disorders are even more likely to run in families than is schizophrenia.

Family studies have consistently shown that the relatives of people suffering from affective disorders have a much higher rate of mania and depression than occurs in the general population. These types of affective disorders do not tend to "breed true"—that is, the relatives of people with bipolar disorder have both bipolar and unipolar disorder, as do the relatives of patients who have depression only. These results suggest that mania and depression may not be two separate illnesses but rather the same illness with different degrees of severity.

In other words, bipolar illness may simply be a more severe form of affective disorder than is unipolar illness.

The rates of illness in relatives vary, depending on the narrowness of criteria used to define the disorder. In general, rates are higher than those reported for the relatives of schizophrenics. For example, about 20 percent of the parents of patients with affective illness also have affective disorders, while the rate in brothers and sisters and children is even higher—possibly as high as 30 percent. The rate tends to be higher in the female relatives than in the male relatives, just as affective disorder is somewhat more common in women than in men. Interestingly, the spouses of people suffering from affective disorder also have a relatively high rate of affective illness—about 20 percent. We are still not sure whether this is because of "assortative mating" (people tending to marry others with similar problems) or because living with a depressed person eventually makes a spouse depresssd.

Twin and adoption studies have also been done for the affective disorders. As in the case of schizophrenia, these studies indicate that genetic factors are important, but that they do not tell the whole story. The concordance rate for identical twins is around 50–60 percent, while the rate for dizygotic twins is 15–20 percent. Adoption studies of affective disorder are still in their early stages, but the preliminary results of these studies also suggest the presence of a purely genetic component that influences the development of affective disorders.

ENVIRONMENTAL AND SOCIAL FACTORS

Common sense tells us that our mood tends to be very sensitive to the things that happen around us. When we experience personal misfortunes, such as the death of a loved one, marital discord and divorce, or misbehavior in our children, we tend to feel sorrowful, discouraged, and despondent. Some people, however, appear to have more natural resilience in recovering from personal disappointment than others do. An inherited lack of emotional resilience may be the predisposing factor—the necessary but not sufficient cause—in the development of affective disorders. This resilience could be programmed in the brain in its neurotransmitter systems, such as the norepinephrine and serotonin systems.

The environmental or social factors that trigger the development of affective illness may be either physical or psychological. Physical stresses might include many different things, such as a minor illness (e.g., a cold), a major illness (e.g., heart disease), or normal fluctuations in body rhythms such as occur during the menstrual cycle. Social factors can include acute stresses, such as a loss or accident, as well as more chronic stresses, such as being married to an alcoholic, living with a disruptive child, or the responsibility of caring for an elderly and infirm parent. Sometimes a series of very small stresses may have a cumulative effect. A dent in a new car isn't much, but when coupled with a violent argument with one's husband and a reprimand from one's boss, it can overwhelm the system, especially if the person is already predisposed to develop depressive symptoms.

The model just described concerning the interaction between social and biological factors has not been proved, but it is widely accepted by many psychiatrists because of its inherent common sense. It fits both the evidence gathered to date from research and the clinical experience of most practitioners. Thus it provides a convenient way of thinking about how depressions are caused or triggered.

What Causes the Anxiety Disorders?

As the "biological era" in American psychiatry began to dawn about fifteen years ago, investigators were quick to explore the brain mechanisms that might play a role in the development of schizophrenia or the affective disorders. The anxiety disorders, however, were relatively neglected until quite recently.

There are several reasons for this relative neglect. First of all, anxiety is a very common human emotion that most of us have experienced, and our experience usually suggests that anxiety is produced by obvious psychological influences. We become anxious when we are about to meet someone important, before we give a speech, before we confront some new and dangerous situation, or before asking a favor of someone. The cause of our unpleasant subjective sensation of anxiousness seems to lie not within ourselves but in our stars. Second, this intuitive sense that anxiety develops in response to environmental threats has been confirmed through the teachings and theories of psychoanalysis. The anxiety disorders have been the principal domain of psychoanalytic research, leading to widely accepted theories that explain anxiety on the basis of psychological factors.

As in the case of both the affective disorders and schizophrenia, it is likely that environmental factors play an important role in producing the anxiety disorders. The relationship between our internal biology and the environment that surrounds us is almost certainly interactive, and it would be foolish to ignore this fact. Nevertheless, recent research has also demonstrated that major biological mechanisms also play a role.

NEUROCHEMICAL FACTORS

Although the antianxiety agents have been in use as long as neuroleptics or antidepressants, investigators have done little to explore their mechanism of action—in spite of the fact that the antianxiety agents are perhaps the most widely prescribed drugs in current use. Annual consumption this year will probably be around 10,000 tons.

The understanding of how antianxiety drugs work was held back until recently by insufficient knowledge about how receptors work and about the GABA system in the brain. The GABA system was mapped somewhat later than the acetylcholine, dopamine, serotonin, and norepinephrine systems. Investigators were aware that it existed and that it probably worked to exert an inhibitory effect, unlike the other classical neurotransmitters, which are predominantly excitatory. We now suspect that one way antianxiety drugs work may be to enhance the effect of GABA, thereby assisting it in modulating or slowing down other brain systems that might be stimulating arousal or anxiety, such as the norepinephrine system. One might think of GABA as the brake in the brain.

While the understanding of how antianxiety drugs might work by assisting GABA has helped us recognize that anxiety might also be localized in the brain, another recent advance has given further support to the neurochemical origins of anxiety. In 1977 several different investigators reported that they had found a receptor site in the rat brain that was especially programmed to receive chemical messages given by antianxiety drugs. They called this site the "benzodiazepine receptor," after the commonest class of antianxiety drugs, the benzodiazepines, which include Valium and Librium.

Like the discovery of the binding sites for the endorphins (or endogenous opioids) a few years earlier, this discovery was met with great excitement. Not only does the discovery give us more information about how the antianxiety drugs work, but it suggests that the brain may have its own inherent receptor mechanisms developed to assist in neurochemical control of psychological states such as anxiety. The benzodiazepine receptors are widely distributed throughout the cerebral cortex, suggesting that they have an important and diffuse modulating effect. Repeatedly, experiments in animals have shown that all types of antianxiety drugs bind to these benzodiazepine receptor sites and that their degree of binding is well correlated with their therapeutic effects. Further, very recent work has suggested that GABA receptors and benzodiazepine receptors tend to be located close to one another on neurons, implying that they may somehow mutually facilitate one another.

This work on the neurochemistry of anxiety is too new to have as yet yielded a well-developed theory concerning the neurochemistry of anxiety. Its most important effect is to make clear that just as the brain contains mechanisms to produce movement or speech, so too it contains mechanisms that are neurochemically encoded to regulate psychological states such as anxiety. During the next several years, the understanding of neurochemical mechanisms underlying anxiety will continue to evolve, and we will begin to understand this important human emotion in terms of chemical processes occurring in the brain.

GENETIC FACTORS

Investigators were also somewhat slow in exploring genetic factors in the anxiety disorders; thus here too research is still in its preliminary stages. Nevertheless, evidence is steadily accumulating that a predisposition to develop anxiety disorders may also be partly hereditary.

Several different family studies of anxiety disorders have now been completed. Very early primitive studies, based on reviews of patients' records and collecting family histories from patients, suggested that the relatives of people with anxiety disorders have an illness rate of about 20 percent, as compared with a rate of about 5 percent in the general population. Female relatives are affected about twice as often as male relatives. More-sophisticated studies, based on interviewing all available relatives, have also been done. When relatives are interviewed directly, the illness rate rises dramatically to about 40 percent, as compared with about 10 percent in interviewed relatives of control subjects. Two twin studies have also been done and have shown a concordance rate of 30–40 percent in monozygotic twins and a rate of 5–10 percent in dizygotic twins. Because of the relatively high MZ-DZ ratio, the twin studies suggest that there may be a significant genetic component to anxiety disorders.

OTHER PHYSICAL FACTORS

For years anxiety disorders were thought to be psychologically caused. Only one lonely piece of research from the 1960s suggested otherwise, and this bit of evidence was left neglected until relatively recently. During the 1960s investigators at Washington University in St. Louis experimented with the effects of giving sodium lactate to people who complained of having anxiety disorder with panic attacks. These investigators noticed that the symptoms of panic disorder were similar to those of hypocalcemia (low blood calcium), and they suspected that patients with panic disorders might have some kind of underlying problem in body chemistry. They knew that the chemical substance lactate tended to reduce blood calcium, so they decided to experiment with using it to produce panic attacks.

The solution was given intravenously and was therefore called the "lactate infusion test." Some people were given "normal saline," a solution containing a mixture of salts similar to that occurring naturally in the body, while others were given lactate. The patients given normal saline noticed no significant effects, but many of the patients given lactate experienced panic attacks during the infusion period. Although the original theory about the mechanism by which lactate produces panic attacks has not been well supported, the experimental technique itself has nevertheless proved useful in exploring physical causes of anxiety.

As interest in biological components of anxiety disorders has reawakened during recent years, investigators have rediscovered the lactate infusion test. They have used it, for example, to determine the best methods for treating panic attacks. One approach has been to compare patients treated with imipramine, a drug thought to be relatively powerful in the prevention of panic attacks, with patients who were untreated. They have found, as did investigators during the

1960s, that lactate infusion produces panic attacks in about 90 percent of untreated patients who complain of having had panic attacks in the past, but it produces no symptoms of panic in control patients. On the other hand, patients with panic disorder who have been pretreated with imipramine typically report no panic attacks. The implication is that imipramine, usually thought to be a drug relatively specific for treating depression, also has important effects in preventing anxiety.

In conjunction with studying the effects of lactate infusion, investigators have also examined changes in neurochemical and neuroendocrine responses. For example, they have explored whether lactate infusion produces major changes in the production of cortisol, prolactin, norepinephrine, and epinephrine. The principal finding noted so far has been that patients who have panic attacks tend to have higher levels of epinephrine, suggesting some abnormality in the catecholamine system. This work is still in its preliminary stages, and it promises to tell us much more about the mechanism of panic attacks in the future. Whatever the results, however, it seems likely that patients who suffer from panic attacks do so because of some type of underlying biological abnormality.

Another very interesting physical problem recently observed in patients with panic attacks is a relatively uncommon cardiac defect known as "mitral-valve prolapse." The mitral valve is one of the four valves that are present in the heart and have the function of preventing blood from leaking back when the heart contracts. The mitral valve is located on the left side of the heart, the side that pumps oxygenated blood throughout the body. Interest in the relationship between mitral-valve prolapse and panic disorder came from the observation that many people suffering from mitral-valve prolapse complained of symptoms similar to those noted in anxiety disorder or panic disorder, such as fatigue, chest pain, pounding heart, shortness of breath, and anxiety.

Since the presence of mitral-valve prolapse is easily determined through a painless and safe technique known as echocardiography, investigators at the University of Iowa have studied a group of patients complaining of panic attacks and a control group. Prior to the echocardiogram, no cardiac abnormalities had been reported in any of the patients with panic attacks. Nevertheless, nearly half the patients with panic attacks had evidence of mitral-valve prolapse on their echocardiograms, as compared with 10 percent of the control subjects. Further, the patients with mitral-valve prolapse tended to have a high rate of panic disorder in their first-degree relatives—about 30 percent, compared to only 4 percent among the control group.

Other investigators have repeated this study and also found a high rate of mitral-valve prolapse among patients suffering from panic disorder. These studies indicate that some patients with this illness may have a physical cause that has gone unnoticed. Doctors might have gotten a clue about the abnormality during routine physical exams by listening to heart sounds, since patients with mitral-valve prolapse have subtle abnormalities such as very soft murmurs and clicks, but typically these are sounds that doctors tend to dismiss as insignificant. It is now clear that some patients who complain of symptoms of panic disorder actually have some type of cardiac abnormality that is producing the symptoms. Consequently, any patient with symptoms of panic disorder should have a thorough set of tests of heart function, including an echocardiogram, an electrocardiogram, and exercise stress test.

What Causes the Dementias?

More is known about the causes of the dementias than about the causes of any of the other major psychiatric illnesses. The causes vary depending on the type of dementia, but all the dementias share the common features of loss of nerve cells in the brain and brain atrophy. Often the loss of neurons can be observed on CT scan, since patients with dementia frequently have ventricular enlargement and cortical atrophy. CT-scan abnormalities are not present in every case, however, particularly early in the illness when the symptoms are still mild. Furthermore, some neuronal loss appears to occur as a natural part of the aging process, and slight evidence of brain atrophy on CT scan may reflect this normal process rather than the development of dementia.

ALZHEIMER'S DISEASE

Technically speaking, there are two types of Alzheimer's disease that differ in age of onset and rate of progression—one called "Alzheimer's disease" and the other "senile dementia of the Alzheimer's type." This distinction is probably arbitrary, however, and so both types are called Alzheimer's disease in this book.

When Alzheimer first described the disease that bears his name, he noted that patients with this disorder had characteristic brain abnormalities that could be seen under the microscope when their brains were studied after death. He observed two abnormalities that stained heavily with a stain containing silver: One was large, dark smudges, which he called "senile plaques," and the other was a scattering of knots that looked like tangled threads, which he called "neurofibrillary tangles." We now know that he was looking at the consequences of neuronal death. In the process of dying, the neurons had more or less exploded, leaving their axons and dendrites behind as the funny knotted mess that he called "neurofibrillary tangles."

Although these changes occur all over the brain, they are most severe in the area of the hippocampus. That probably explains why memory loss is a prominent symptom of dementia. As was described in chapter 5, the capacity to learn and remember resides in several different parts of the brain, but removal of a single major center on both sides can lead to profound memory loss. Scoville's famous patient, H.M., who was frozen in an eternal present and totally unable to remember any new information that he was given, got that way through having his hippocampi removed surgically on both sides of the brain.

The abnormalities in Alzheimer's disease can be seen at the microscopic level, but they are associated with another abnormality occurring at the neurochemical level. In this instance, the deficiency appears to be in the cholinergic system, which is widely distributed throughout the cerebral cortex and the subcortical gray-matter regions. Patients with Alzheimer's disease show clear evidence of a decrease in cholinergic transmission. It is not yet clear whether the deficiency in acetylcholine occurs everywhere in the brain or is localized in some small but important area such as the hippocampus or the subcortical nuclei, which have an important function in memory and cognition.

Alzheimer's disease has also been observed to run in some families, but it is not yet clear whether this is due to genetic factors or to some other cause, such as infection with a viral agent. An unusual type of virus that remains dormant for a long time and therefore produces quite delayed effects (known as a "slow virus") has been identified in one extremely rare illness leading to dementia—Jakob-Creutzfeldt disease. Thus Alzheimer's disease could be caused by either hereditary or environmental factors or some mixture of both.

MULTI-INFARCT DEMENTIA

Multi-infarct dementia is another relatively common form of dementia. Although similar to Alzheimer's disease in that it produces memory loss and other signs of intellectual deterioration, it differs in its clinical course and in its cause. Multi-infarct dementia is due to a series of small strokes occurring over an extended period of time. Although no single stroke is extremely serious, the cumulative effect is great. Sometimes the strokes are accompanied by obvious symptoms, such as mild paralysis or aphasia. At other times the strokes affect parts of the brain with less-obvious functions and often pass unnoticed as "silent strokes." Nevertheless, a CT scan may show small areas of abnormality where brain tissue has died due to loss of its blood supply.

Multi-infarct dementia illustrates how the causes of a disease can be explained at many levels. At the simplest level, one can say that multi-infarct dementia is caused by a series of small strokes, which in turn are caused by some factor that cuts off blood supply to the brain, usually the buildup of sludge and clots in the arteries and their small branches that supply blood to the brain. At another level, this disorder is caused by the various factors that predispose to the development of clogged blood vessels anywhere in the body. The same factors that predispose to a heart attack also predispose to stroke. These include high blood levels of cholesterol, possibly a high-cholesterol diet, smoking, insufficient exercise, and high blood pressure, to mention only a few. Furthermore, strokes and heart attacks also tend to run in families, so there may be an underlying genetic predisposition. As in the case of schizophrenia, the explanation of the causes turns out to be "multifactorial."

HUNTINGTON'S CHOREA

Huntington's chorea is a very rare type of dementia that is worth noting primarily because its causes are relatively well understood on many different levels. Huntington's chorea runs in families and, unlike affective disorders or schizophrenia, it has a clear Mendelian mode of transmission. While most mental illnesses are probably caused by a complex interaction between environmental and genetic factors, Huntington's chorea is almost purely genetic. When one asks what causes Huntington's chorea, the answer is therefore perfectly clear: It is caused by genetic programming that is built into the DNA that forms the genes which are part of the nuclei in the cells of our bodies. Traits programmed on genes have several different patterns of transmission that are considered "classically Mendelian," after the patterns originally observed by the Austrian monk Gregor Mendel when he bred peas in his garden.

The pattern of transmission in Huntington's chorea is autosomal-dominant. Forty-four of our chromosomes are autosomal (i.e., determine the nonsexual characteristics of our bodies), while the other two are the X or Y chromosomes that determine our sexual characteristics. The autosomal chromosomes govern the remainder of our body characteristics. These chromosomes form twenty-three pairs, and only one set of twenty-three chromosomes is passed on by each parent to the offspring through an egg or sperm. To say that a gene is "dominant" means that the trait it carries always dominates over the opposing gene in the pair. A person who has Huntington's chorea has one dominant gene that dictates developing this illness, while the opposing gene is weak or neutral in this respect. When two people have children, each child receives half of each parent's genetic material. If one parent has Huntington's chorea and a child is unlucky enough to get the set of chromosomes carrying the gene for this disease, then that child too will develop the disorder. Putting the matter another way, the child of a person with Huntington's chorea has a fifty-fifty chance of developing the disease.

Although Huntington's chorea is rare, what makes it dreadful is that the disorder usually does not become apparent until middle age. By the time people recognize they have Huntington's chorea, they have already gone through the childbearing years and passed the illness on to their children. People from families with Huntington's chorea must live with a painful double uncertainty: They must live thirty or forty years wondering if they will develop this dreadful dementing illness, and they must wonder whether they might meanwhile be passing this illness on to their children. Alternatively, they must decide whether to risk having children.

When Huntington's chorea eventually strikes, its symptoms are similar to those of other dementias. The person becomes confused, forgetful, irritable, and socially inappropriate. In addition, patients with Huntington's chorea tend to develop severe depressive symptoms and may also develop psychotic symptoms such as delusions. Further, there are obvious physical symptoms such as muscular twitches and facial grimacing. Within the brain, the illness manifests itself through deterioration of the basal ganglia, particularly in the caudate nucleus. This can often be seen on CT scan, since the caudate appears quite small and the frontal horns of the ventricles are enlarged.

Psychiatrists are particularly interested in Huntington's chorea because it provides a useful model for understanding the brain mechanisms that may be involved in other types of mental illness. In this instance, we have very specific knowledge about what causes the disease, both in terms of how it is transmitted and the part of the brain involved. Damage to a relatively small part of the brain, and a part once thought to modulate only motor activity, in fact produces a wide range of symptoms, the most serious of which involve our ability to think and feel.

10

QUO VADIS?:

A Better Future

To lighten the affliction of insanity by all human means is not to restore the greatest of the divine gifts; and those who devote themselves to the task do not pretend that it is. They find their sustainment and reward in the substitution of humanity for brutality, kindness for maltreatment, peace for raging fury; in the acquisition of love instead of hatred; and in the acknowledgment that, from such treatment improvement, and hope of final restoration, will come if hope be possible. It may be little to have abolished from the madhouse all that is abolished, and to have substituted all that is substituted. Nevertheless, reader, if you can do a little in any good direction—do it. It will be much, some day.

—CHARLES DICKENS,
"A Curious Dance Around a Curious Tree"
Household Words, January 1852

Shortly before Christmas of 1851, Charles Dickens paid a visit to Saint Luke's Hospital for the insane in London. By this time the hospitals had been "reformed": William Norris and the other chained inmates had disappeared. Although Dickens could no longer feel moral indignation about how the mentally ill were treated, his social conscience was clearly touched by the injuries that mental illness itself produced. Although physical chains were gone, the mentally ill were still in the bondage of a crippling disease. He described what he saw in a Christmas essay, "A Curious Dance Around a Curious Tree," which ended with the plea to his readers quoted above. It remains an appropriate plea today.

Today, however, doctors can do much more to lighten the affliction of insanity than they could in 1852. Much of that progress has been described in this book. What are the causes and implications of this progress, both bad and good, for the present and future? How can the reader of today, if he or she chooses to try, "do a little in any good direction"?

Mental Illness and Moral Responsibility

One obvious implication of the biological perspective in psychiatry, stressed throughout this book, is that the mentally ill—and their families—no longer must carry a burden of blame and guilt because they have become ill. While episodes of illness are sometimes triggered by unfortunate life events, the basic causes lie in the biology of the brain. The best way to treat these biological abnormalities—treatment that is not always available at present—is to correct the underlying physical abnormality, usually through the use of somatic therapy.

Some readers may feel strong intuitive objections to this implication, even those who recognize that it is far more humane than to assume that the mentally ill are possessed, self-indulgent, or just plain lazy. It seems a bit extreme to imply that the mentally ill may have *no* responsibility for becoming ill or for remaining that way. If they have no responsibility, are they not then given a license to do as they please? Isn't this dangerous for society? How should someone who must deal with an ill relative or friend react to the illness? Isn't it better to expect the ill person to do something to help himself?

Of course the mentally ill have some responsibilities. While a person suffering from depression or schizophrenia may not be able to help the fact that he has this illness, it benefits neither him nor society to treat him as if he is a helpless and irresponsible cripple. The advantage of the biological perspective is that it removes stigmatization of, and anger toward, the mentally ill. It would do them a disservice if it completely removed the sense of mutual obligation to one another and society that we all share as part of the human condition.

If mental illness is a physical illness, then patients, doctors, family members, and society should all behave toward a patient just as they would if he had cancer or heart disease. As stated earlier, if a person has had a recent heart attack, we never feel he has "brought it on himself" (even if common sense tells us that he may have in part by smoking or eating too much or failing to exercise). But once he has suffered the attack, we usually expect him to take part of the responsibility for getting better. He should slowly begin to exercise regularly, should lose weight as needed, and should take medications as prescribed. Some heart-attack victims are unable to return to work, but most can; a very few use their illness as an excuse for malingering. Most heart-attack victims confront their rendezvous with death with courage and stoicism, but a few use it as an excuse for self-pity or attention-seeking. Sometimes it is hard to tell whether the heart-attack victim is using his illness to manipulate, but in such cases we usually give the person the benefit of the doubt.

Likewise, most people who are mentally ill recognize that they have a problem, and they want to get better. Most seek treatment voluntarily and comply reasonably well with medical advice. Most would like to be able to return to work, and in fact most do so. The healthiest way to approach the future prospects of a depressed or anxious person is to assume that he will get better and resume an essentially normal life. Even though his illness may be biologically caused, just as is a heart attack, that does not free him from an obligation to seek treatment, comply with it, and to love and to work like everyone else. Some patients with severe schizophrenia or dementia will become totally incapacitated, just as happens to people with severe heart disease. For them we should have the same compassion that we all have for other human beings who are very sick.

What If a Patient Refuses Treatment?

If the mentally ill have a social obligation to seek and comply with treatment, what should one do about those who refuse treatment? Although we find it painful and irritating, we all recognize that a person with cancer has the right to refuse treatment and even to die. Do the mentally ill have the same right to refuse treatment? In this situation the patient with schizophrenia or some other serious mental illness may differ from the cancer patient in one important way: The person with cancer has the right to refuse treatment, *assuming he is able to make the decision rationally.*

Sometimes a person in the midst of an episode of illness, particularly an illness such as mania or schizophrenia, is not able to make rational decisions. Such people may be forced to obtain treatment against their will, otherwise known as "commitment" since the treatment is usually administered in a hospital setting. Laws about commitment vary from one state to another, but most stipulate that a person can be made to accept involuntary treatment only if he is dangerous to himself or others.

The definition of *danger to self* often evokes considerable controversy. Should it be applied narrowly and refer only to physical danger, such as suicide? Should it be applied more broadly and cover the possible consequences of impaired judgment, such as social or financial indiscretions and dangers? Who is to judge dangerousness, and how should it be judged? The answers to these questions are not always easy. Some states place the burden of decision on judges and lawyers, with the great disadvantage that people within the judicial system know little about medicine and may err excessively in the direction of either overprotecting the patient or feeling a need to punish him for misconduct. On the other hand, when decisions about requiring treatment are in the hands of doctors, concern is aroused that their self-interest is served. After all, doctors may find it economically advantageous to require treatment, or they may be excessively protective and paternalistic toward the patient because trying to cure the ill is ingrained in them as a part of their training.

Thus, there are no simple answers from the law on the issue of when treatment should be required for the mentally ill. From the point of view of friends and relatives, it is usually best to try to convey trust in the medical system to the patient, so that he will seek treatment voluntarily. Nevertheless, patients can and should sometimes be forced to obtain treatment against their will if they are very ill and do not recognize it.

Are All Mental Illnesses Biologically Caused?

This book has concentrated on four classes of serious mental illnesses that are at least in part biologically caused: the affective disorders, schizophrenia, anxiety disorders, and dementias. What about other common disorders, such as alcoholism, drug abuse, and personality problems?

These disorders have not been discussed in this book because we know much less about them. A few clues suggest that at least some of them may also be partially due to biological causes. Alcoholism, for example, tends to run in families, which may or may not suggest a genetic component. Many people who abuse alcohol and drugs may also have significant problems with anxiety and depression, and in fact their tendency to abuse these substances may sometimes be secondary to a biologically based affective disorder.

Some types of personality problems—variously referred to as "schizoid," "schizotypal," or "borderline"—have been shown through twin and adopted-offspring studies to have a genetic relationship to schizophrenia or the affective disorders. One researcher has done a study of criminal behavior and its associated personality disturbance, which is characterized by disregard for social and legal norms (called "antisocial personality"). He examined adopted children born to female criminals in state penitentiaries and found that these children, although adopted immediately and reared within normal families, tended to have a much higher rate of criminal conviction than did the adopted offspring of normal mothers, suggesting that even antisocial personality may have a biological component.

The implications of this latter study are rather frightening, for they suggest that genes may control far more of our destiny than has usually been suspected. Most of us tend to assume that criminal behavior is due to a host of social factors, such as poverty, poor parenting, and inadequate education. Only when those of us who are parents recall how children seem to have enormous differences in personality from the time of birth—patterns that often seem to evolve autonomously no matter how we try to shape them—do we confront the possible realization that even our personalities and social behavior may be in part genetically programmed into our brains from birth.

Does the Biological Revolution Lead to Biological Determinism?

The psychodynamic perspective seemed to take destiny out of our own hands and place it in the hands of those who shaped us during the first few years of our lives: Seductive or authoritarian fathers and smothering or schizophrenogenic mothers taught us patterns of reacting that could be quite difficult to escape. Psychodynamic theory implies a psychological or social determinism: We become what we are through an interaction between instinctual drives and early life experiences, both of which are largely outside our control; our free will enters the picture only when, as adults, we decide to learn new techniques for dealing with the consequences of these shaping forces.

The biological perspective seems to replace one type of determinism with another, which may seem even more awesome and overwhelming. The biological perspective implies that mental illness is largely due to factors outside the patient's own control, primarily to the type of brain and body he was born with and the environment in which they have been nourished. While this perspective may seem deterministic, it is not totally so. In the first place, neuroscience also stresses the notion of "plasticity"—that is, the brain has built into it the ability to adapt and change in response to injury or to changes in the environment. For example, while language is usually "built" into the left hemisphere, children who have substantial damage to the left hemisphere early in life still learn to speak quite normally; the brain recognizes the injury and develops new ways for language to develop in the remaining parts of the brain. Even adults who have had strokes are often able to overcome their disabilities in speaking or walking.

While identity and personality undoubtedly do reside somewhere within our brains and are at least partly programmed there from birth, we feel as if they are separate and under our control. Living our lives with our own particular assigned brains is like playing a game of cards with a particular hand that we have been dealt. We cannot control the cards we are given, but we can choose how we will play them.

What About the Genetic Pool?

The biological perspective suggests that the tendency to develop mental illness is at least partly determined by genetic factors. This, too, is a kind of determinism. What implications does this have for the individual and society?

At a personal level, people who themselves have some type of mental illness or who come from families with mental illness must feel some concern about passing the tendency on to their children. Some may even wonder whether they should have children at all. In general, this is a false concern for several reasons. First, common mental illnesses such as depression or the various anxiety disorders are no more incapacitating than many other illnesses that are also at least partially familial, such as cardiac disease. If people chose not to have children because of a family history of medical illness, few of us would procreate. Second, as the previous chapter has shown, genetic factors only partly account for the development of mental illness. Even identical twins, with exactly the same genes, are concordant only about half the time. Other personal and environmental factors also clearly play a major role. The only serious disorder for which genetic factors appear to be preeminent is Huntington's chorea, and this is the only mental illness that might contraindicate having children.

There is a serious risk that people may overemphasize the importance of genetic factors in mental illness. While these factors clearly influence the development of illness, we still do not know precisely to what extent or how. The rates of illness in relatives, described in chapter 9, are not very high. Providing a good environment through preventive medical measures such as good hygiene and good nutrition may turn out to be much more important than genetic factors. Hitler's Germany, more on the basis of intuition than scientific data, urged that the mentally ill be sent to the ovens in order to purify the race. A professor on a medical-school admissions committee once argued that we should obtain a family history of mental illness from all applicants in order to prevent the admission of students predisposed to mental illness. Hitler's Nazis and the professor of medicine both possessed a dangerous and fanatical knowledge: They knew not what they knew not, and they wished to make decisions about others' lives using only a tiny kernel of fact. Mental illness, like many other illnesses, is partly influenced by genetic factors. But genetics are only a small part of the story. Family history of mental illness does not predict that particular members of the family will become ill; in fact, the odds are relatively low. The mentally ill do not contaminate the human genetic pool. Indeed, some illnesses, such as the affective disorders, may be associated with traits that benefit society, such as energy, intelligence, and creativity.

Will the Biological Approach Dehumanize Psychiatry?

Despite its occasional obvious foolishness, the discipline of psychiatry has also filled a useful and important niche. While the rest of medicine has devoted itself to making great technological advances, the role of psychiatrists has often been to teach other physicians that they must talk to patients as people, learning how to imaginatively reconstruct different individual reactions to the experience of illness.

They have reminded other doctors that they must try to understand each patient within the context of her social, economic, and family environment, so that treatments would not be prescribed that the patient could not afford, or could not understand, or could not accept for personal or religious reasons. Until recently, the psychiatrist was the only kind of doctor left who could be guaranteed to spend more than ten or fifteen minutes talking to a patient. If psychiatry becomes more medical and biological, will not its humanizing influence on the rest of medicine and its concern for the patient as a person be lost?

One hopes not. Even with the development of improved treatments and some laboratory tests, psychiatry is likely to remain a relatively humanistic specialty, at least in the hands of good practitioners. For although the biologically oriented psychiatrist may believe that he is treating a disorder in the brain, its symptoms appear in the way the patient thinks, talks, feels, and relates to others. Psychiatrists will have to remain sensitive to these processes, and no doubt they will continue to remind their colleagues of their importance. Further, even with improved technology, psychiatry will continue to require that doctors spend substantial amounts of time with their patients in order to assess the subtle and complicated symptoms of mental illness and the impact of these symptoms on the patient's life.

To some extent, the humanism of psychiatry will be ensured by the process of self-selection. Most medical specialists choose a particular discipline because they find it interesting or challenging to them personally. They choose psychiatry because of an interest in the mind or brain. (As the life history of Freud indicates, it is but a small jump from the brain to the mind and back again. The jump to the liver or gallbladder is much larger.) People usually go into psychiatry because they want to understand what makes people tick, mentally and emotionally; because they are curious about the causes and effects of mental illness; and because they want to try to help those who suffer from it. Contrary to popular belief, psychiatry is the lowest paid of all the medical specialties, and it also tends to be the lowest in prestige. Presumably, people must choose this field simply because they like it.

Will Psychotherapy Disappear?

Not likely. First of all, some people are going to continue to want this form of treatment, and where there is a demand, there will be a supply. For some people, having a listener who is neither friend nor family fills a void that could not be filled in any other way.

Further, psychotherapy is probably the preferred treatment for some types of problems. While self-esteem or excessive guilt may be abstract concepts that in fact refer to neurochemical processes in the brain, we have no idea where they reside, nor any inkling of how to modulate them chemically. On the other hand, psychotherapists have been modulating these abstract concepts through listening and counseling for many years and have developed well-established techniques for doing so.

Even the most biologically oriented psychiatrist would not deny, if pressed, that a mental illness such as depression can wreak havoc with a patient's personal or social life. While the patient may require a somatic therapy to correct an underlying chemical imbalance, he may also need psychotherapy to deal with the personal and social consequences of his illness. He may need help with his marriage, with learning to find a new type of work, or simply with learning to live with the fact that he has had an episode of mental illness. In many cases, psychotherapy and somatic therapy will work hand in hand.

Over the years, however, the popularity of psychotherapy for very mild problems may diminish, and intensive psychotherapy will almost certainly be used less frequently for serious mental illnesses. Psychotherapy is costly in terms of both time and money. As insurance companies try to place a ceiling on the rising costs of health care, elective psychotherapy for mild problems is an obvious place to cut. When patients find themselves paying the entire bill, they may find intensive psychotherapy to be a luxury they cannot afford. Intensive psychotherapy has not proved to be a very effective treatment, especially in isolation, for the serious mental illnesses, even though less-frequent supportive therapy may be helpful. Consequently, its popularity has already decreased markedly. It is also likely that for many patients brief psychotherapy will be combined with monitoring of somatic therapies and will sometimes be compressed into shorter appointments, often lasting only fifteen minutes.

As the fifteen-minute appointment replaces the fifty-minute hour for many patients, they may actually find it preferable after they recover from their initial surprise. Briefer appointments are a more efficient and economical way of providing psychiatric care for a larger number of people. Frequently, patients have minimal or no insurance coverage for outpatient care, and are relieved to have briefer, less expensive appointments if they are sure it is adequate. Much of the time, fifteen minutes is long enough for doctor and patient to talk to one another about the patient's symptoms and how they are affecting his personal life. A decrease in the quantity of time spent does not necessarily mean a decrease in the quality of the care provided.

Can Mental Illness Ever Be Cured Through Biological Techniques?

The word *cure* is used much too liberally today. We need to learn to distinguish between cure and care. People have been too often taught by both physicians and journalists to hope for "a cure" when in fact they should be hoping for care instead.

Very few diseases are actually cured, and even cures usually leave a few scars. Infections can often be eradicated completely by antibiotics with no later signs that the illness has occurred. Surgical repair of hernias or removal of diseased organs sometimes leads to improvements so striking that they could be called a "cure," although there is always a scar. But most illnesses are managed rather than cured. The diabetic is treated with insulin, with considerable benefit, but this does not constitute a cure. The patient with Parkinson's disease improves markedly on L-dopa, but she is not cured. The patient with coronary-artery disease is relieved of chest pain through nitroglycerine, but the clogged arteries that prevent adequate nourishment from reaching the heart and therefore cause pain cannot be opened up. The pain and inflammation of arthritis can be decreased, but not eliminated. And so on for most diseases, including the mental illnesses.

The somatic therapies sometimes produce an improvement so striking that it appears to be a cure. This is particularly the case when depression is treated with tricyclics. But although the episode of depression may be cured, the tendency for the illness to recur remains, and therefore even this is not really a cure. Mania and the anxiety disorders also respond well to medication, but sometimes recur. For schizophrenia, there is help, but there are no miracles, and we are still seeking a good treatment for dementia. A true cure would totally eliminate the symptoms of these diseases and also prevent recurrence. Although we lack a cure, which can only come when we fully understand the mechanisms causing the illness (and perhaps not even then), improvements in care have dramatically ameliorated the condition of mental patients during the past twenty-five years.

How to Help?

A reader who has persisted to this point must care enough about mental illness to wonder what he or she can do to help the plight of the mentally ill. Obviously, the first step is to do everything that can be done to eliminate the stigmatization of mental illness. Society must come to view it as a type of disease like any other, not as something to evoke fear or shame. Mental illness should not be treated like a skeleton in the closet. When people begin to talk about mental illnesses openly and freely, this will do much to lessen prejudice against mental illness.

Increased knowledge about mental illness should also help a great deal. As law courts, social-service agencies, employers, and schools begin to realize that mental illnesses are not all the same, they will be able to react more sensitively and intelligently to particular people suffering from mental illness. A person with an anxiety disorder or a depressive disorder, for example, can usually be expected to return to normal levels of functioning with adequate treatment. People suffering from mania also typically return to full normality, except for the uncommon instance where a person suffers from many repeated severe episodes of mania, especially beginning at a young age. The main problem that friends and associates of manic patients must confront is that the manic individual is often reluctant to seek treatment, although obviously she should be encouraged (and even sometimes forced) to do so. People with these disorders cannot and should not be deprived of their jobs, their places in school, or their professional credentials. There is a wide range of possible outcomes for patients with schizophrenia, and their illness must always be dealt with on an individual basis.

Friends and associates of a person who has had a psychiatric illness often wonder how to react. They do not want to embarrass the person by indicating that they know about his problem, and many are afraid that they might even make him worse by bringing it up or referring to it. A person who has had mental illness may of course wish to keep the fact a secret, particularly as long as he must fear being blamed or shamed, but most would welcome a friendly acknowledgment that they have been ill, especially if it is accompanied by a gesture of friendship or goodwill, such as an invitation for a drink, dinner, or a theater engagement. Like Bill in chapter 1, patients often feel embarrassed and guilty about having been ill, and this situation is worsened when their friends and associates ignore the problem or avoid them.

A second way to help is to nurture psychiatric research in every way possible. People contribute generously to the Heart Association or the Cancer Foundation, and they are roused to peaks of emotion and generosity by telethons for muscular dystrophy. There is no Mental Illness Foundation, nor are there telethons for the mentally ill. (In fact, it is ironic that the chief federal institute for research in mental illness felt obliged to euphemistically call itself the National Institute of Mental Health rather than the National Institute for Mental Illness.) The biological revolution may eventually mobilize psychiatrists and the general public to form large public foundations similar to the Cancer Foundation to help support the search for causes and treatments of mental illness.

Even without such large-scale efforts, however, people can help in small ways. Patients and their families can participate in research programs whenever they are asked. The knowledge that we already have about the causes and treatments of psychiatric illness could only have been obtained through the generous cooperation of patients and their families. People who have thought about donating organs, such as eyes or kidneys, should also consider donating their brains to one of the "brain banks" being set up for research in mental illness. Since we must understand mental illness through exploring its underlying causes in the brain, and since it is still difficult to study the brains of people while they are alive, postmortem brain research offers a powerful tool for unlocking many of the secrets of mental illness. These brain banks need a group of normal brains so that they can make comparisons with those of patients suffering from mental illness. Patients who have mental illness may also contribute a great deal by willing their brains to these brain banks.

Quo Vadis?

If we compare the world of today to the world of William Norris or even of Dickens, we can see that we have made great progress. The psychodynamic perspective has awakened interest in the mind and in mental illness, reducing fear and prejudice substantially. The introduction of a biological perspective will reduce it even more. The coming years promise revolutionary advances in the field of psychiatry, in both the medical and social spheres.

Medically, we can expect that the exciting growth in neuroscience research will continue to bear rich, varied, and useful fruits. Within the past ten to twenty years, the neurochemistry of the brain has been carefully mapped, much as the neuroanatomy was in the late nineteenth century. We know that there are both chemical and structural breaks in the brain in several types of mental illness. During the coming years, these will be charted in increasingly fine detail. As we grow to understand causes, we can find better ways to prevent or to treat. The technology for studying the brain in living people, such as CT scanning or PET scanning, has been available for less than ten years. This technology is moving ahead at breakneck speed. As they improve and become more accurate, these imaging techniques and other laboratory tests for mental illness will become part of standard medical practice during the coming years, thereby improving the precision of diagnosis and assisting in the search for causes. Research in neuroscience tends to cross-nurture: Advances in neurochemistry will lead to advances in neuropharmacology, so that we can also expect the development of new and better somatic therapies. Psychiatry today is much like general medicine forty or fifty years ago—on the brink of discovering its own version of insulin, penicillin, blood transfusion, and cardiac pacemakers.

Socially, we can hope for a new era of enlightenment about mental illness, similar to that of the classical Greeks. Because mental illness is so common, striking the friends and relatives of nearly all of us (or even us), we can ill afford to hide it under a blanket of ignorance. Once they are armed with information and knowledge, those friends and relatives can become participants in a renaissance of interest in and concern for mental illness. In the future, society itself must march, not to the asylum, but to the streets and marketplaces where we all live in order to free the mentally ill from the chains of social opprobrium and misunderstanding. In the future, Bill and others like him will be spared.

Glossary

Affect A term used in several different ways and therefore somewhat confusing. In the context of affective disorders, affect usually refers to mood—an emotional state that tends to vary in response to stimuli and situations. In the context of schizophrenia, the term "affect" tends to refer to the general capacity to experience any emotions. Thus the schizophrenic who has lost his capacity to feel and express emotions normally is said to have affective blunting or affective flattening.

Affective disorders Mental illnesses characterized principally by abnormalities in mood. The two principal classes are mania and depression. Manic disorder is characterized by euphoria, accompanied by other symptoms such as decreased need for sleep, pressured speech, racing thoughts, grandiosity, and poor judgment. Depressive disorders are characterized by low mood, usually accompanied by insomnia, decreased appetite, poor concentration, loss of interest, and diminished ability to experience pleasure.

Afferent neuron A nerve cell designed to carry messages into the brain from various kinds of sensory receptors, such as those in the ears or the eyes. An *efferent neuron* is designed to carry messages out of the brain in order to command parts of the body to perform some action, such as commands to muscles to move.

Agoraphobia Literally, fear of the marketplace. This type of mental illness is manifested by an extreme fear of venturing out, usually away from the patient's home. Often agoraphobia is accompanied by panic attacks—unpleasant overwhelming episodes of anxiety accompanied by pounding heart, tremulousness, and shortness of breath.

Akathisia A side effect of neuroleptics characterized by an unpleasant sensation of internal restlessness and physical manifestations such as pacing or restless movement of the legs.

Akinesia Diminished motor activity. This symptom is common in schizophrenia and in disorders affecting the basal ganglia, such as Parkinson's disease, as well as injuries to some parts of the frontal system.

Alogia Diminished capacity to think or to express thoughts. This is a common symptom of schizophrenia. It expresses itself clinically through a tendency to speak very little or, even when speech is relatively normal in amount, to say little in terms of content. The speech tends to be over-abstract or over-concrete.

Antipsychotic drugs Drugs designed to diminish psychotic symptoms, such as delusions or hallucinations. These drugs are also referred to as neuroleptics. They were also once referred to as "major tranquilizers," although this term has now been largely abandoned.

Aphasia Impairment of the ability to communicate verbally, caused by damage to the language centers located in the left hemisphere. There are many different types of aphasia; the symptoms vary depending on the portion of the language center that is affected. For example, Broca's aphasia is characterized by difficulty speaking and poor articulation, but with intact comprehension; the injury is located in the anterior part of the language center. Wernicke's aphasia is caused by damage to the posterior regions of the language center and is characterized by impaired comprehension and abundant but nonsensical speech.

Autosomal dominance A pattern of genetic transmission. Forty-four of our 46 genes are autosomal; that is, they govern physical characteristics other than sexual characteristics. (The latter are controlled by the two non-autosomal chromosomes, the X and Y chromosomes, that determine whether we are male or female.) Our physical characteristics are programmed on various parts of the chromosomes that are referred to as genes, with each gene carrying information for different traits. Chromosomes are paired, with half coming from each parent. If a gene on one chromosome is more powerful than its opposing pair, it is said to be dominant. Only one dominant gene need be present for the trait to be expressed. On the other hand, some traits are said to be recessive. In this instance, the trait must be present on both gene pairs in order for the trait to appear. Huntington's chorea is an example of an autosomal dominant disease, while hemophilia is an example of an autosomal recessive disease. Diseases located on the sex chromosomes are said to be "sex-linked." Color blindness is an example of a sex-linked disorder.

Avolition A symptom of mental illness that is particularly common in schizophrenia. This symptom is expressed as extreme apathy and loss of normal drive and interest. An avolitional patient often finds it difficult to get started at tasks or, if he begins a task, often gives up before he has finished it.

Axon The part of the neuron that carries messages from the cell body to nerve terminals or synapses. Axons are wrapped in a fatty substance, the myelin sheath, which makes them appear lighter; therefore parts of the brain composed principally of axons are called white matter. The cell bodies of neurons are located in areas such as the cortex or subcortical structures such as the caudate or thalamus. Since the cell bodies are darker in appearance, they compose the parts of the brain referred to as gray matter.

Basal ganglia Specialized regions of gray matter located inside the brain that include the caudate and putamen. Because of their appearance in cross-section, parts of the basal ganglia are also referred to as the striatum and the lenticular nucleus. The basal ganglia are modulators of movement and integrators of sensory information. Because they are rich in dopamine, they are often affected by neuroleptic drugs, which have major effects on the dopamine system. For a schematic, *see* figure 7.

Behaviorism A scientific point of view that argues that the best way to understand the human mind and personality is through the objective observation of behavior rather than through subjective introspection. Behaviorism tends to stand in firm opposition to the psychodynamic point of view, since the latter stresses the importance of internal subjective experience.

Bipolar disorder A type of affective disorder characterized by episodes of mania. Most bipolar patients experience both poles of affective disorder, or both mania and depression. A few experience only mania; by convention, these patients are nevertheless referred to as bipolar. Bipolar disorder is equivalent to the older term *manic-depressive illness.* Patients who experience only episodes of depression are usually referred to as *unipolar.*

Cerebral cortex ("bark of the brain") Up to six layers of neuronal cell bodies that cover the surface of the brain. Because of the dense packing of cell bodies, this part of the brain appears darker when examined visually in cut sections, and therefore it is often referred to as gray matter. Different parts of the cortex are highly specialized and control different functions, such as vision, language, or recognition of spatial relationships. The activities controlled by this part of the brain are sometimes referred to as "higher cortical functions." The cortex is much more highly developed in man than in any other animal.

Chromosome A portion of the cell nucleus that codes genetic information. For further description, *see* Autosomal dominance.

Cingulotomy A form of psychosurgery that involves cutting a small portion of the cingulate gyrus (a part of the limbic system). Performed very infrequently, this is the only type of psychosurgery in current use. It is performed principally in cases of obsessive-compulsive disorder or depression that are extremely incapacitating and have not responded to any other form of therapy. Cingulotomy has supplanted the older procedures of prefrontal lobotomy and prefrontal leucotomy, both of which involved cutting rather large white matter tracts in the frontal region as a treatment for schizophrenia.

Commissurotomy A surgical procedure that involves cutting the corpus callosum. This procedure has been done in an attempt to relieve the symptoms of patients who have intractable seizures. Since this surgical procedure cuts the white matter fibers that connect the left and right hemispheres, patients who have been "commissurotomized" have been studied by neuroscientists in order to understand the functional capacities and relationships of the two hemispheres.

Corpus callosum ("tough body") The white matter fiber tracts that connect the left and right hemispheres.

CT scan Computerized tomographic scan (also referred to as CAT scan, or computerized axial tomographic scan). This is one of several "brain imaging" procedures currently used to study brain structure in living human beings. The brain is X-rayed, and computerized techniques are used to reconstruct relatively precise pictures of brain structures. Prior to the development of CT scanning, it was only possible to examine calcified structures such as bone using X-rays.

Delusion A fixed false belief. Delusions involve believing things that are not there, while hallucinations (*see* below) involve seeing or hearing things that are not there. Delusions are frequently persecutory (believing that one is being conspired against), grandiose (believing that one has special powers), or somatic (believing that one's body has been changed or damaged).

Dendrite Branching processes that extend out from the neuronal cell body and enlarge its capacity to receive messages from other neurons.

Disconnection syndrome A syndrome that results when the white matter tracts connecting two command centers are disconnected from one another through some sort of damage, such as occurs in a stroke.

Dizygotic twins Twins who come from two different eggs or ova (di = 2, zygote = egg). Twins of this type are usually referred to as non-identical or fraternal, and they are genetically equivalent to siblings. Because they come from two different fertilized eggs produced by the union of two different sperms with two different eggs, and because the sperm and the egg contain the 46 chromosomes that dictate our genetic development, dizygotic twins are genetically quite different. On the other hand, *monozygotic twins* are produced when a single fertilized egg divides (for reasons not yet known) and begins to evolve into two separate but genetically identical individuals. Thus monozygotic twins have essentially identical genetic material.

Double-blind trial   A type of drug trial in which both the patient and the investigator are ignorant as to which drugs the patient is receiving. Usually an experimental drug is compared to a placebo, or to an already established drug, or (ideally) to both. Because both the clinician and the patient are "blind," this type of trial produces the most scientifically objective results.

Dysphoria   An unpleasant or uncomfortable mood state, such as depression or anxiety, contrasted with *euphoria,* the mood that characterizes manic disorder.

ECT   Electroconvulsive therapy. This form of treatment involves applying a small amount of electrical current to the patient's temples, after the patient has been put to sleep and given a muscular relaxant. The electrical current produces a seizure, which occurs only in the brain because the muscle relaxants keep the body from reacting. The therapeutic mechanism of ECT is not known, but it is recognized as a highly effective treament for depression. It is used much less frequently in either mania or schizophrenia.

EEG   Electroencephalogram. A technique for measuring the electrical activity of the brain. It is a painless procedure that involves applying a network of electrodes to the surface of the head using a salty jelly similar to that used for an electrocardiogram. These electrodes are connected to a machine called a polygraph, which records squiggly lines that reflect the electrical activity of various parts of the brain. EEGs are used to help diagnose seizure disorders, brain tumors, disorders in metabolism, damage produced by head injury or drugs, and abnormalities in sleep patterns.

Efferent neuron   A neuron specialized to send out messages. *See* Afferent neuron.

Extrapyramidal system   A brain system that assists in the regulation of motor activity. It exists parallel to (and relates with) the principal motor system (the pyramidal system). This system consists principally of the basal ganglia (*see* above). Because neuroleptic drugs have important side effects due to their actions on the extrapyramidal system, these are sometimes referred to as "extrapyramidal symptoms." Such symptoms include akathisia, stiffness and rigidity, and tremor.

Gene   A part of the chromosome that regulates a particular body function.

Generalized anxiety disorder   A disorder characterized primarily by free-floating anxiety. When anxiety is also accompanied by attacks of panic (pounding heart, shortness of breath, etc.), then the more specific term "panic disorder" is used.

Glial cell   "Glue cells." Glial cells are small neurons that are specialized to provide nourishment and support for the command neurons located in gray matter regions such as the cortex or the basal ganglia.

Gray matter   Areas in which large neuronal cell bodies are relatively densely packed. These areas are located principally in the cortex and in subcortical regions such as the thalamus or caudate. Since they have a dark appearance in cut section, they are referred to as gray matter.

Hallucination An abnormality in perception. Most hallucinations experienced by psychiatric patients are auditory; they involve hearing various kinds of voices. More rarely, hallucinations may involve seeing things, tasting things, or feeling things that are not in fact there (*see* Delusions).

Hypothalamus The region of the brain located just below the thalamus. The hypothalamus is a major regulatory center that relays messages from other parts of the brain to the pituitary gland, the command center for neuroendocrine functions.

Limbic system A set of related structures that regulate emotions, memory, and perhaps aspects of attention. Parts of the limbic system include the cingulate gyrus, the septal region, the fornix, the mammillary bodies, etc. The limbic system is particularly rich in dopamine. For a schematic picture of the limbic system, *see* figures 5 and 6.

Manic-depressive An older term now rarely used, but roughly equivalent to bipolar (*see* Bipolar disorder).

Motor homunculus A figure drawn in order to show which parts of the brain control movements in various parts of the body. The motor homunculus shows that some parts, such as our hands and our faces, occupy large regions of the brain, while others are controlled by relatively small areas (*see* figure 9).

Multi-infarct dementia A type of dementia produced by numerous small strokes. Many of the strokes may be so minor that they even pass unrecognized, while a few will be marked by motor symptoms such as paralysis or difficulty in speaking. As a consequence of these repeated strokes, the patient begins to show progressive intellectual deterioration.

Neuroanatomy The study of brain structure.

Neurochemistry The study of how messages are communicated through neurons by various chemical transmitters.

Neuroendocrinology The study of the way the brain regulates endocrine systems in the body, such as the adrenals, thyroid, ovaries, or testes.

Neuroleptic drugs Drugs used principally to regulate the symptoms of psychosis. They are also known as antipsychotic drugs.

Neuron Nerve cell.

Neuropharmacology The study of the way that various drugs may affect neuronal and brain functions.

Neuropsychology The study of cognitive, perceptual, and volitional systems in the brain, with an attempt to localize these functions as precisely as possible.

Neurosciences A group of related disciplines that attempt to understand how the brain works under normal conditions and how these normal functions can be damaged through injury or disease. Basic neurosciences include neuroanatomy, neurochemistry, neuropsychology, neuropharmacology, and neuroendocrinology. Psychiatry and neurology are the clinical medical specialties that examine the abnormalities produced by disease.

Neurosis In classic psychodynamic theory, a disorder caused by psychic conflict. In more recent use, the term "neurosis" refers to milder disorders such as the anxiety disorders or mild depression. Sometimes it also refers to disorders that make the patient feel uncomfortable and therefore are called "ego dystonic." Because the term has multiple meanings and is therefore unclear, some psychiatrists have suggested that it be abandoned as a way of classifying mental illness.

Neurotransmitter A chemical messenger that one neuron uses to communicate with another. Many different types of neurotransmitters have been discovered in the brain during the past several decades, and many more are currently in the process of discovery. Some of the best known include dopamine, norepinephrine, serotonin, acetylcholine, and GABA.

NMR scan A scan done by nuclear magnetic resonance. This new type of scanning procedure involves the use of magnetism rather than radiation. The patient is placed in a chamber and a large, powerful magnet is turned on. The magnet exerts a force on certain substances in the patient's body that are sensitive to magnetism, and so they move in response. When the magnet is turned off, the elements relax to their original position. Because different parts of the body contain different concentrations of these substances and therefore move to different degrees, the amount of movement can be used to reconstruct a picture of organs in the body, such as the brain. Unlike CT scanning, NMR does not involve the use of radiation. Like CT scanning, it is painless. As in the case of CT scanning, computerized methods are used to reconstruct the pictures obtained. NMR may give clearer pictures than CT scanning, although at present it takes somewhat longer to complete a scan.

Opiate receptors Receptors on neurons that are specially programmed to receive messages from opiate-like substances such as heroin or codeine. During recent years, it has been discovered that the brain contains its own endogenous opioids (the endorphins) that interact with these opiate receptors.

Panic disorder A type of anxiety disorder characterized by panic attacks—sudden bursts of anxiety accompanied by a sense of impending doom and a variety of physical symptoms such as pounding heart and shortness of breath.

PET scan Positron emission tomographic scan. A brain imaging procedure that involves the use of positron-emitting substances that are injected into the body and taken up by the brain. The radiation that they emit is measured and used to construct a picture of the brain. Unlike CT or NMR, PET scanning is a "dynamic" procedure. That is, it permits the study of brain function in addition to brain structure.

Phobia An irrational fear. When this irrational fear is excessive or incapacitating, a person is usually said to have a phobic disorder. Common phobias leading to disorders include agoraphobia (*see* above) or social phobias such as fear of speaking or of eating in public.

Placebo "I shall please." A substance not known to have any active medicinal properties. Sometimes in the past, placebos were given to patients with persistent complaints that were not thought to have any medical foundation; a substantial number of these patients responded to the placebo, and the result is referred to as a "placebo effect." The use of placebos is considered unethical in modern medicine, except in the context of a drug trial. In such trials, the goal is to determine whether a new experimental drug is better than a placebo. When they participate in these trials, patients are told that they may receive an active drug or a placebo.

Post-traumatic stress disorder A type of mental disorder occurring in people who have experienced a stressor outside the range of normal human experience, such as death camps, natural disasters, or mass catastrophes. Symptoms include persistent reliving of the experience, a feeling of psychological numbness, and prominent symptoms of anxiety and depression.

Prefrontal leucotomy   A surgical technique that involves cutting of white matter tracts in the prefrontal regions. Originally developed as a treatment for schizophrenia, this procedure is no longer in use. It has sometimes been referred to loosely as "prefrontal lobotomy." It has been largely supplanted by cingulotomy (*see* above).

Pseudodementia   A syndrome in which the patient shows many of the symptoms of dementia, but does not in fact have a genuine dementing illness such as Alzheimer's disease. Perhaps the most common pseudodementia syndrome occurs in patients suffering from severe depression. They may manifest memory impairment, disorientation, and apathy, and yet these symptoms disappear completely when the depression is fully treated.

Psychiatrist   A medical specialist trained to practice psychiatry. Most psychiatrists have completed four years of medical school and four years of residency training in psychiatry, including some training in neurology as well. Psychiatrists vary widely in orientation, some taking a biological approach, others a psychodynamic approach, and others striving to be eclectic and balance all relevant approaches.

Psychoanalyst   A therapist who specializes in psychoanalytic psychotherapy. Most psychoanalysts are psychiatrists, although there are also a few "lay analysts" who are not physicians. Most analysts have gone through medical school, a psychiatry residency, and analytic training, which involves a personal analysis. Narrowly defined, psychoanalytic psychotherapy involves the use of a couch and treatments occurring four to five times per week. More broadly defined, psychoanalytic psychotherapy involves the use of psychodynamic principles and theories. The narrow concept is sometimes called psychoanalytic psychotherapy; the broad concept is referred to as psychodynamic psychotherapy.

Psychologist   A person trained in psychology. Most psychologists have obtained a master's degree or a Ph.D. in psychology. Some have also completed a postdoctoral internship in which they have had experience treating patients. Psychologists involved in patient care are usually referred to as clinical psychologists. Psychologists can provide psychotherapy and behavioral therapy, but since they do not have medical training, they cannot prescribe medication.

Psychosis   A term, like neurosis, that has multiple meanings. In its most precise definition, it refers to illnesses characterized by "psychotic symptoms" such as delusions or hallucinations. Sometimes the term is used more loosely to refer to disorders that are severe or incapacitating, such as schizophrenia, mania, or serious depression.

Psychotherapist   A person specializing in the use of psychotherapy, a treatment technique that involves listening and talking to a patient, helping her develop insight about her psychological mechanisms, and teaching her to overcome maladaptive mechanisms. Psychotherapy may be practiced by psychologists, social workers, psychiatrists, and the clergy. Some states have relatively restrictive licensing laws that define who may perform psychotherapy, while others have essentially none.

REM sleep   Rapid eye movement sleep. This type of sleep is shown on EEG by large lines reflecting rapid eye movements. It represents the periods during sleep when a person is dreaming.

Schizophrenia   A type of mental illness characterized by prominent psychotic symptoms such as delusions or hallucinations, as well as other symptoms such as disorganized thinking and speech, loss of volition, and affective flattening. Many psychiatrists believe that schizophrenia is in fact a group of several different disorders that vary in symptoms, response to treatment, and outcome. Thus schizophrenia is sometimes subdivided into good prognosis *versus* poor prognosis schizophrenia, positive *versus* negative schizophrenia, paranoid *versus* nonparanoid schizophrenia, etc.

Skinner box   A cage specially designed to study how giving various rewards or punishments can affect the behavior patterns of rats. Because the box was designed by Skinner, one of the foremost proponents of a behavioral approach to understanding human activity, the Skinner box has become a symbol of the behavioral approach.

Synapse   The junction between two neurons across which chemicals (neurotransmitters) are sent to permit one neuron to communicate with another. Many of the drugs used in psychiatry appear to work by modulating chemical transmission at the synapse, and consequently many psychiatrists hypothesize that the abnormality in these disorders is neurochemical in nature.

Tardive dyskinesia   A movement disorder produced by long-term intake of neuroleptic drugs. Its manifestations include writhing and twitching movements of the face and sometimes of other parts of the body.

Thalamus   A gray matter region located deep inside the brain that is clearly visible on CT scan. The thalamus serves principally as a modulatory relay station to integrate information from and send messages out to other parts of the nervous system.

Tricyclic antidepressant   A type of medication used principally for treating depressive illnesses. There are many different types of tricyclics. Some of the more common are Elavil, Tofranil, Norpramin, Aventyl, Vivactyl, and Sinequan. These drugs are referred to as tricyclics—their basic chemical structure contains three rings.

Ventricular system   Four fluid-filled structures inside the brain. Their function appears to be to cushion and nourish. They contain cerebrospinal fluid. Because they appear vividly on CT scan, they serve as important landmarks. When parts of the brain have atrophied, the ventricles often enlarge to compensate; therefore they serve as important indexes of brain atrophy.

Wernicke's aphasia   A type of aphasia caused by damage to the posterior language area in the left hemisphere (Wernicke's area) and manifested by abundant productive speech that is nonsensical and by inability to comprehend the speech of others.

White matter   The portion of the brain composed principally of axons. Its appearance is somewhat lighter than the regions composed of neuronal cell bodies, since the myelin sheath surrounding the axons makes the tissue appear lighter. Because this contrast is clearly visible on cut sections, these areas are referred to as white matter.

Index